SILENT VICTORY

SILENT VICTORY

BY CARMEN McBRIDE

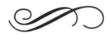

With a Foreword by

Albert W. Knox, Ph.D., *Chief, Audiology and Speech Pathology Service Kansas City Veterans Administration Hospital*

And an Introduction by

Donald E. Kuenzi, M.D.

NELSON-HALL COMPANY • CHICAGO

Library of Congress Catalog No. 73-84602
Copyright © 1969 by Carmen McBride

Nelson-Hall Co., Publishers, 325 W. Jackson
Blvd., Chicago, Ill. 60606

Manufactured in the United States of America

To Ben

Contents

Preface

Silent Victory was my husband's idea. When the stroke left him with aphasia, he could not accept his loss of speech, but kept pointing to his mouth, asking, Why? Why did this have to happen to me?

Then one day he wrote the word "BOOK" on a pad and pointed to me and to himself.

"You want us to write a book," I asked, "about our experiences?"

He did.

"If we could have found such a book in 1956 — or now — we know how much it would help us," I said.

He agreed.

As we started to keep notes for the book, I remembered our reading in a medical journal about a doctor with aphasia who misspelled "hospital" much the same as Ben did. That gave us a feeling of kinship.

When Ben started to write notes for the book with his left hand, I knew he wanted me to tell the aphasic who had lost the use of his right hand to learn to write with his left hand. By writing, even if he is limited to single words often misspelled, he can communicate. If he loses both speech and writing, he may retire into himself, feel that he no longer is good for anything and were better off dead.

The book was one project we were not able to finish together. In fact, we accomplished very little. It was too tiring for Ben.

That is the reason I wrote *Silent Victory* — for Ben, for the hundreds of thousands of aphasia victims, and for their families.

Foreword

Mrs. McBride has written of the experiences she and her husband had in conquering the emotional obstacles and interpersonal barriers which cause major problems in recovery from aphasia. Her work is well worth reading and studying. For the scientist and the clinician she has answered a most important question, specifically, "Is a good and full life possible when there has not been much recovery of the losses of communication skills?"

The McBrides were fortunate, because out of their misfortune they were able to build happiness and contentment into their lives. Many times I have seen the opposite of this story unfold where the question was "How can a patient recover his language if the only things he has to talk about are so overwhelmingly unpleasant that he is unable to face them?"

The scientist and clinician were both caught short by aphasia. Until recent times patients with severe strokes did not live long enough to come to the attention of the speech pathologist. Those patients who did survive were not understood. Nobody knew what to do for them.

The entire field of aphasiology has come into existence

11

subsequent to World War II. At that time new medical procedures were introduced. Now patients not only recover, many take their place in society and the economic world. As a result, those of us who interact with those patients on a daily basis found ourselves charged with the responsibility of accumulating a body of scientific information and recording the results of experimental, historic, environmental, and clinical studies. We have hope that many of these research procedures will lead toward recovery from aphasia.

Many laboratories and clinics in universities and hospitals are directing their efforts to the aphasia recovery problems. Some of us are engaged in experimental studies directed toward understanding how aphasic patients learn and what avenues of learning and stimulation are the most productive or the least frustrating. Other groups are working toward understanding attitudes which predispose the patient toward recovery or toward dependency, that is, whether the patient makes the effort to recover or just gives up. Many are working to arrive at accurate descriptions of the patients' symptoms and hope to develop predictions on the basis of successive performances on examination tasks.

While the outcome of the experimental efforts are unknown, it is safe to say that the future is brighter than the past. The advent of teaching machines, computers, and other electronic aids to instruction utilizing programs of language recovery which have been found to be effective, and utilizing the modern principles of reinforcement in learning developed by our colleagues in psychology has enabled us to provide, more realistically than ever before, an environment in which recovery can occur.

This is what a speech pathologist does: He isolates the communications difficulty confronting the patient. He provides an atmosphere in which recovery can take place, he provides stimuli designed to precipitate or enhance the recovery process, and he provides an attitude of his own which serves to keep the patient on the path of recovery until his optimum level is achieved.

Albert W. Knox, Ph.D.
Chief, Audiology and Speech
Pathology Service, Kansas City
Veterans Administration Hospital

Introduction

The telephone rings. A familiar voice says, "Something is the matter with my husband. He awakened this morning and was unable to speak, or to move his right arm or leg."

These are all too familiar words in the life of today's primary physician. The diagnosis is not difficult. The patient has had a stroke — or a cerebral vascular accident — or in abbreviated terminology, a CVA.

Should the loss of speech (aphasia), or loss of function of the arm and leg (hemiplegia) be permanent, the medical, psychological, economic, and social implications for the affected person and his family are staggering. Fortunately, a goodly number of people so affected will recover some or all of the impaired functions, either through the passage of time, the efforts of medical personnel, or the intelligent and loving care of a devoted family.

Today's medical doctor, who practices general or adult medicine, is seeing an increasing number of cerebral vascular accidents. This is a direct result of increasing longevity in our population, and the attendant arterial

15

disease which accompanies advancing age.

Strokes in younger age groups (below 50 years) are quite unusual. They are generally the result of the rupture of a congenitally weak or malformed blood vessel (artery) deep in the brain circulation, or of a blood clot (embolism) which becomes dislodged from a diseased heart and goes to the brain. Brain tumors and brain infections (abscesses) also may cause stroke.

In older age groups, the causes of stroke center largely around the process of hardening of the arteries — arteriosclerosis — although modern investigative techniques are showing that other causes are also important. At least one-third of stroke-like illnesses occurring in older age groups can be attributed to causes other than arterial hardening, such as brain tumor, rupture of a congenitally weak blood vessel in the brain as in younger people, brain injury resulting from a traumatic blow to the head, or spread of a cancer to the brain from elsewhere in the body.

Approximately two-thirds of strokes in older age groups occur as a result of arterial hardening. One-half of this number occurs because of narrowing of major arteries in the neck — an area which may well be surgically accessible. The other half occurs because of narrowing and plugging of small arteries in the brain itself. These groups have a common causative factor — arteriosclerosis — or atherosclerosis — or hardening of the arteries.

Newer diagnostic techniques have given new hope of help for the already developed stroke. No longer is pessimism the rule when a person develops symptoms of a stroke-like illness. The doctor's first thought in such an instance is to find out as nearly as possible the exact classification of the stroke. Is it due to hemorrhage, cerebral thrombosis (a blood clot in a brain artery), a closing off of a neck artery due to the atherosclerotic process which in turn denies the brain needed blood supply and oxygen? Or might it be due to a brain tumor, brain infection, the consequences of an injury, a blood clot coming from another source such as the lungs, or perhaps a result of metastatic spread from a distant cancer?

To find more specifically what caused the paralysis, speech loss, mental confusion, or unconsciousness, with which the patient presents, today's doctor will set in motion a series of diagnostic tests in a step-wise manner. A spinal tap, skull x-rays, electroencephalogram (brain wave test), pneumoencephalogram (air contrast x-ray of the brain), and finally cerebral arteriography (x-rays of the blood vessels of the brain accomplished by injecting a dye into the arterial system), might all be performed before a proper diagnosis can be made.

Once a satisfactory, definitive diagnosis is established, treatment becomes much more selective. The neurosurgeon may have much to offer if the problem proves to be a brain tumor, or a leaking blood vessel which is surgically accessible, or more commonly, a narrowing or closing off of one of the vital neck arteries which supplies the brain with blood.

For these strokes which have caused paralysis or speech problems (aphasia), and are not amenable to surgical correction, there is a great deal to be done from the standpoint of rehabilitation. The family physician, physical therapist, speech therapist, occupational therapist, and, most of all, devoted family members, may all be utilized to obtain maximum restoration of function. The problem of aphasia, in particular, requires the most careful and correct handling by family members and close contacts. An intelligent, speechless person can indeed be helped to find satisfactory methods of expressing himself if those about him understand his problem, and assist in appropriate ways.

A large portion of the medical researchers' efforts has been directed to diagnosing and treating the accomplished stroke. Great strides have been made. But the real thrust of present and future efforts must lie in stroke prevention — which in large measure means the prevention of hardening of the arteries. Much has already been done in arteriosclerosis prevention. Significant medical studies have been made the past several years linking the cause of arteriosclerosis to such elements of health as diet, thyroid function, estrogen lack in women after the menopause, and smoking.

If the practicing physician is going to make these discoveries meaningful and helpful to his patients, he must advise starting the preventive program early in life. Ideally this would be when the person was in his twenties — before the hardening process starts.

In older age groups, where arteriosclerosis is already present, very effective medical means of slowing this process are already available. The older person who is noticing transient dizzy or blackout spells, loss of balance, lapses of memory, unusual headaches, intermittent slurring of speech, or brief periods of numbness of arm and leg should have a careful physical and laboratory examination, so that the necessary preventive steps might be taken. Every adult in our population should have regular yearly physical exams, with selected laboratory studies such as blood cholesterol and triglycerides, blood sugar determinations to rule out diabetes, and tests for thyroid function.

Arteriosclerosis prevention will mean a somewhat less palatable diet for many persons who have a tendency toward diabetes, or high blood cholesterol, or triglycerides. It will mean early detection and control of hypertension, and avoidance of obesity and smoking. Later, in the fifth decade, and after, it might mean a diagnostic x-ray of the blood vessels which feed the brain. It may mean increases in physical activity. For post menopausal women it may mean taking estrogenic substances which are known to give protection against development of arteriosclerosis. Supplemental thyroid hormone might be advised.

The accomplished stroke, with permanent residual paralysis or aphasia, is an awesome problem for the patient and his family. A hopeful note here, is that, if all the presently known techniques of stroke prevention could be applied to our adult population, the frequency of this devastating and perplexing affliction could be greatly reduced.

Donald E. Kuenzi, M.D.

~ 1

The Stroke – Aphasia

"Ben, you are a bigger man now than ever," a friend said to my husband that night at the dinner. Ben looked at her and shook his head. I knew he was saying, "Can't you see I'm done for?"

She did not hear him. No one in the room heard him. Ben had lost his speech. This was our first appearance socially since the stroke left him with aphasia — loss of speech, writing, reading, spelling and figuring.

For the forty-one years of our marriage, we had worked together building the life of our dreams. It did not seem possible that in one blow our world could be shattered.

Saturday, January 7, 1956, the day of the stroke, had been happy. Ben no longer went to his employment agency office in Kansas City on Saturday but that morning by telephone from home, he had set up an interview for a salesman. Twenty-nine years of finding employment for people made him confident that the applicant and the employer were right for each other.

That afternoon, we had met the builder who was to start the exhibition ranch house in Lawn Acres, our twenty-three acre subdivision, five miles from our small

21

farm home in Kansas City North, Mo. We had chosen plans and from the exhibition house hoped to sell lots and build more houses.

It was five o'clock when we returned home. As we left the car in the basement garage, I said, "Hungry?"

"Starved," Ben answered.

"In that case shall we forget the steak we did not take from the freezer and settle for hamburgers?"

"No," he said. "Let's make it a picnic."

"All right. You start the charcoal and I'll get the steaks."

I went to the freezer for the steaks. Ben stayed in the basement to open a new sack of charcoal. We would meet at the picnic grill. Ten minutes later when I saw that he was not at the grill, I went to the basement and found him on the floor. The stroke.

He had had a heart attack and three other strokes. The first stroke left no disability. The second, only a slight weakness in the right hand and arm. The third left him with loss of vision to the left in both eyes. Later, we had managed that. When he drove the car, I watched to the left for him.

I looked at him now as cold and gray as the cement floor on which he lay. I must get blankets and a pillow, but first I had to telephone Dr. Harrison Trippe and our daughter, Nancy.

"Please lie still, dear," I said on the chance that he might hear me. "I'll be right back." When I returned he had not moved.

Nancy and Harvey, our son-in-law, who lived on a small farm twelve miles from us, were there in minutes. By the time the ambulance came, Nancy and I had Ben's bag packed and the house ready to close. Harvey had wrapped the blankets around Ben and stayed with him.

At the hospital, Dr. Trippe had a private room and a special nurse waiting for us. Ben soon had oxygen. The nurse and I sat beside his bed all night . . . the longest night I had ever known. It did not seem possible that only hours ago, he had been so full of life, so happy. He was not suffering. That was a comfort. But how would he feel when he realized what had happened to him? If he thought he was going to be crippled for the rest of his life, would he lose his will to live? It was hard to imagine him without his willpower. I had seen it turn many crises into victory. If he did lose it, would I be strong enough to help him regain it?

It was more a prayer that a question. And I realized that I had been praying from the moment I found Ben on the basement floor. I closed my eyes and repeated now . . . "God is our help in every need." When I opened my eyes and looked out of the window, there was the dawn of a new day. I was no longer afraid.

Ben was moved to group nursing that morning. He had had around-the-clock nurses two years before and we knew what they could do for him. But never had they worked as they did now. Oxygen and so many other tubes, I didn't know what they all were for. I did know that he was getting the best care possible.

He did not move. He made no sound. I watched him through the day and when night came, I knew I could not leave him to go home. I arranged to close the house indefinitely and leave our dog with a neighbor, and then rented a small apartment near the hospital. We had no cattle on the farm that needed care as we had sold the steers we had pastured through the summer. Now I could be with Ben every day, from early to late.

At first, after he regained consciousness, he showed no interest in his surroundings. Just when he realized that he was in the hospital, I do not know. I saw him looking at me, asking: what happened?

I drew my chair close to his bed. "You have had a stroke, dear," I said, "but already you are better." He studied my words and tried to move his right leg. When he found he couldn't, he shook his head. "It will be all right in a few days," I said. "That other time you lost the use of your right side, it came back in a few days."

I saw that he was trying to move the big toe of his right foot and I said, "Try again."

It barely moved. "Oh!" he said. His first word since his, "Let's make it a picnic." He smiled and said again . . . "Oh!" . . . just to make sure that he could do it again. But when he tried to say something else and all he could say was, "Oh," I saw fear in his eyes . . . the same fear that was lead in my heart. Had he lost his speech?

Before he could guess my thoughts, I walked over to the dresser, picked up a vase of red carnations and took them to him. When I showed him the card, he didn't try to read it but let me know he wanted me to.

I read it and showed him other flowers and cards that had come for him. "Oh, oh," he said, and I thought he wanted me to read the cards. When I started to read, he shook his head and pointed to his mouth. He was asking, "Why can't I talk? Why can't I say anything but 'Oh?'"

I walked back to the dresser and replaced the cards, then took time to rearrange the flowers. What could I tell him? I was so happy to hear his *first* "oh," it had not occurred to me that it was all he had. When I could trust my voice, I said, "As you grow stronger, your speech will become all right. Sometimes, it takes a little while."

He made no effort to answer. I could only hope that he was not remembering the one person we knew who had lost his speech in a stroke. It had been two years and he still was not able to talk. "When Dr. Trippe comes tomorrow, we'll ask him about your speech," I said.

He was waiting for Dr. Trippe the next morning. He looked at me and pointed to his mouth, reminding me of my promise. Dr. Trippe explained: "Sometimes there is damage from a stroke that affects those parts of the brain which are important for the interpretation of language. The impairment is not unusual. Sometimes it lasts only a few days."

Ben wanted to hear more. I asked Dr. Trippe, "Do you have other patients who have a speech loss?"

"Not right now," he answered. "There is a man down the hall who had a stroke three weeks ago and lost his speech. It has started to come back."

I saw hope light Ben's eyes and said, "When it is all right with you and for this man, we will try to meet him." Ben's smile told me how much it would help just to meet someone else who had lost his speech, and was regaining it.

That night, alone in my apartment, I did a lot of thinking. What was being done to help people who had lost speech in a stroke? There must be books about stroke patients who had lost their speech. As soon as I could leave Ben long enough, I would go to the library and book stores.

But in 1956, I found few books about strokes that I could understand. Everything was too technical. I bought the one book that I thought I might understand well enough to explain to Ben what happened to a person when he lost his speech from a stroke, and what was being done to help him.

"Aphasia." I had never heard the word and didn't know what it meant until I read . . . "Aphasia refers to all aspects of language loss, not only speech. The patient may have difficulty in speaking, reading, writing, spelling and figuring . . . also in understanding what is said to him." Not Ben, I thought. He understands everything that is said to him and he knows what he wants to say. But all he can say is, "Oh!" Why?

There was so much I must learn. And so little time. I could not read at the hospital because I had not told Ben I had the book. When I returned from my leave, I had told him that I had not found anything at the library. I couldn't tell him I had bought the book until I found something in it that would encourage him. So far, all that I had read would only confuse him.

So my reading was limited to evenings at the apartment after nine o'clock. By that time, I was so tired I fell asleep while reading . . . and often dreamed about aphasia. Writing, reading, spelling and figuring — besides speech. Ben was too weak to try writing. He hadn't tried to read his cards. Spelling and figuring — no telling when we would know about them.

Always in the morning, things looked brighter. While I ate breakfast, I read . . . "Aphasias differ in severity from mild to complete. No two are alike." Ben's must be mild, I told myself. He was more alert each day. And with his faith, willpower, and natural ability, he will talk again, I told myself.

I remembered his mother telling me that he had started to talk in public when he was so young that they had to stand him on a table to give his recitations at the meetings of the Literary Society in the country school house. Later in school he had won oratorical contests, and all his business life had been based on his salesmanship.

The morning that the nurse said, "Ben, we're going for a walk down the hall today," he shook his head. "You're ready," she told him. "Remember how well you walked from your bed to the chair yesterday?"

He made a motion as if he were falling. "I won't let you fall," she promised. I knew what he was thinking . . . he'd feel like a fool leaning on her one hundred pounds.

"But I am going, too," I said. His eyes said: my hundred and two pounds wouldn't be much help.

The nurse and I laughed. "Our total of two hundred and two pounds beats your one hundred and sixty-five," I challenged. He grinned and we knew we had won.

It was only about a hundred feet from his room to the sunroom. With the nurse at his right side and I on the left, we started down the hall, Ben wearing his new robe and a smile. By the time we reached the sunroom, his smile had faded. He was so tired that we all sat down to rest. "Tomorrow, it will be easier," I said. Each day was to be better.

The morning when Dr. Trippe said, "How would you like to try a little writing today?" Ben pointed to his mouth, asking, "When can I begin speech therapy?"

"We'll work on speech later," Dr. Trippe told him. "Let's see how well you can write your name. One of these days you may receive a lot of money and you'll have to sign for it."

Ben smiled and pointed to the pencil and pad on his bedside table. When I gave them to him, he dropped the pencil. "He was right-handed," Dr. Trippe said. "Try the left hand." The best Ben could do with either hand was a short, crooked line.

A week later when our lawyer brought papers giving me power of attorney, Ben still could not write his name. I will never forget the look in his eyes when he made his "X" on the signature line and watched the lawyer print "His" above the "X", and below it . . . "Mark." Then on the left side of the "X," the lawyer printed . . . "Ben B." . . . and on the right, "McBride." Under the "Witnesses to the Mark," two nurses signed.

From that day on, Ben and I practiced writing every day. He was so pleased with his progress, he showed it to his night nurse. Whenever she had a little free time, she helped him. Their eyes were shining that morning when Ben showed me his signature. Not the free flowing script of the old days, but bold and clear . . . "Ben B. McBride."

"You're back in business," I told him. "As soon as we can, we'll go to the bank and you can sign a new signature card."

As he continued to write, every letter was printed, with the exception of his "a" and "e." He printed single words only: Usually nouns but occasionally a verb; adverbs and adjectives, rarely; prepositions and conjunctions, never.

The builder called one morning about starting our ranch house. I promised to talk with Ben and phone him. I knew I could not put it off any longer, but what should I say to Ben? If he wanted to go ahead with the exhibition house, how could I tell him he was not able to take on the responsibility of a sales program?

As I watched him write his name again, I was glad that he had mastered one problem before I presented him with another. Finally I said, "Mr. Gentry (the builder) phoned this morning. He wants to know when he can start our house."

Ben laid down his pencil and looked at me. Did I dare to ask, "How would you like to lease the farm and move to Lawn Acres?" No. If that was to be our decision, it must come from him.

I was glad when he picked up his pencil. It gave me more time. Carefully he printed, "LAND ACRE." It had to be "Lawn Acres." He looked up to make sure I followed him, then printed, "HOURSE." "House," I said. Was he telling me that he wanted to go ahead and build the exhibition house? Could I help him sell it and carry on with the sale of other lots ... perhaps build more houses?

While I was thinking how to answer him, he pointed to the words he had just written, "HOURSE" and "LAND ACRE," then to me and himself. "You mean," I said, "that you want to lease the farm and move to Lawn Acres?"

He nodded.

"Wonderful!" I agreed. "I'll love living in a brand new ranch house. Only I hope you won't sell it before we're settled."

His smile told me that was just what he meant to do.

"We'll have to stay until we build another house. It will make it easier for us if we're living over there while we put in the rest of the streets and the utilities. When shall I phone Mr. Gentry?"

He made the motion of snapping his thumb and forefinger.

"Now?"

He nodded.

"If it takes ninety days to build the house, we will have

time to lease the farm," I said. "Shall I ask Mr. Gentry to bring the plans so you can see them again?"

He wasn't listening. Was he thinking about moving from the farm? He was unhappy about something. I started to say, "We'll lease the farm for a year, then move back." But would he be able to go back in a year? We could not plan a year ahead. All we could do was to live a day at a time. I said, "I'll ask Mr. Gentry to bring us the contract." The next day the contract was signed. The house was to be started at once.

Ben's walking and writing continued to improve. But by now, I knew we had a lot of work to do on spelling. Even in short words, the letters were often wrong or transposed. When I tried to correct his mistakes, he was confused. Or he would try so hard, writing the word over and over, I was afraid he would become exhausted. Often the word was so misspelled, I had no idea what it was.

When he pointed to his mouth, I knew he was asking about his speech but there was nothing I could tell him. I had not been able to locate a speech clinic.

He wanted to know about the man down the hall who Dr. Trippe had said was regaining speech. I had learned that his progress was slow and what he said was hard to understand. Sometimes when he wanted to say, "No," he said, "Yes" . . . or "No" for "Yes." There wasn't anything I could tell Ben to encourage him.

I had heard about another stroke patient in the hospital with a speech loss. Allen Smoot. I met his wife in the hospital cafeteria. Allen Smoot was regaining his speech — with problems.

Lila Smoot's eyes filled with tears as she said, "He gets so mad at me, he would strike me if he could. I can't understand it. He was always kind and gentle."

I was thankful that I could tell her that I had just read that in some cases of aphasia that was what happened. A person who had always been kind and considerate would become so frustrated when he couldn't speak, he would strike out at those he loved best.

"But that is not all," she said. "He never used profanity and now, out of the clear, he will say, 'Jesus Christ!'"

Again I could quote from my book, "Automatic speech accounts for the speech of some aphasia patients. They are able to say some fixed expression like . . . 'How do you do?' . . . 'That's okay' . . . or they may swear."

I still don't understand," she said.

There was so much that neither of us understood, we had lunch together as often as we could. Her husband was younger than Ben and had been a foreman at a manufacturing company. She was a secretary in a downtown office and was worried about how she was going to take care of her husband and keep her position. They had to have her salary.

I, too, was concerned about our future. Until Ben could spell better, I dreaded trying to talk to him about it. Would he want to sell the employment agency or would he want to hire someone to run it for him? I was grateful that we had a prospective buyer for the agency.

The morning that he opened the newspaper to the "Help Wanted" ads and turned to "Employment Agencies," I knew he wanted to talk about our employment agency.

A few weeks before the stroke, Ben had been surprised and pleased when Elmer Behrens made an offer for our agency but he had asked for time to think about it. Common sense told him that he should slow down. The employment business, Lawn Acres and the farm, much as he enjoyed them, were too much. He would soon be sixty-five. But finding employment for people and supplying firms with personnel had been his life for so long — perhaps in another year he would sell? If he had a buyer. Or should he sell now while he had an offer?

At just what point in his thinking, the tentative contract had been written, I did not know. I was grateful that it had been written and agreed to by Elmer Behrens and Ben. Our copy was at home.

Ben was still looking at the want ads when I said, "Elmer Behrens has been keeping in touch and wants to talk with you as soon as you feel up to it."

He reached for a pencil and wrote, "CONCART." I didn't know what he meant. He tried again, "CONCERT." "Concert," I repeated to myself. We had said nothing about music. "CONCART," he wrote again. "Contract," I said.

He smiled and patted the pocket of his pajamas, then pointed in the direction of home. "It's still at home," I told him. "In the inside pocket of your brown coat. When do you want me to get it?"

His thumb and forefinger told me, "At once." I got the contract. Mr. Behrens had his lawyer look at his copy. I took our copy to our lawyer. In a few days the deal was closed. When I gave Ben the check, I said, "Cash in full."

He looked at the check a long time; I knew something was wrong. "It is for the amount you agreed on," I said and named the figure.

He still looked at the check. Finally he gave it back to me. I didn't know if he was accepting it because he thought it should have been for more and didn't know how to tell me or had he lost understanding of figures?

I was afraid to suggest that he write the amount that he thought the check should be for. If he could not write it, he would be more confused than ever.

He was making progress in writing words but there was practically no improvement in spelling. If he had lost figuring, too — ? For a man who had been excellent in figuring and spelling — and now without speech — ? Just how much frustration could he take?

Every day seemed to bring new trials and disappointments. There had been the day when he wanted a certain soft drink. The nurse and I finally learned that it was something to eat or drink. But what? When I gave him his pencil and notepad, he shook his head and closed his eyes. We were still trying to figure what he wanted when he opened his eyes and looked out of the window. I will always remember his smile as he pointed to a sign on the drug store window across the street. It advertised the name of the soft drink he wanted. *

It was the next day that the nurse brought good news! The name of a speech clinic. I telephoned for an interview for Ben.

After six weeks in the hospital, Ben was to be dismissed on Sunday. On Monday, a cab would take us to the speech clinic.

Dr. Trippe asked us to stay at the apartment I had rented for a week before we returned to our farm home.

My brother and I were at the hospital at nine that Sunday morning. Ben was walking the hall waiting for us. He pointed to a news item in the morning paper. The daughter of a friend had been in a car accident. But she was not injured, I read with relief.

Ben's smile told me that he, too, was happy for her

* *Together* magazine, November 1963

escape. When he pointed to the news item again, I knew he wanted to make sure that I understood he had regained reading.

He was walking, writing, reading and learning to spell ... and tomorrow the speech clinic. We were making progress.

↵ 2

Hope - First Speech Clinic

When the cab driver left us at the speech clinic, Ben and I stood on the sidewalk looking at the building. I knew we were thinking together: how many other men and women have gone through those doors into a strange, new world of beginning again?

Another cab stopped. The driver and a woman helped a man out of the cab. He walked with a cane and was wearing an ankle brace fastened to his shoe. As we stepped back to let them pass, Ben and the man smiled at each other. The woman said, "My husband is happy to be walking again after his stroke."

"We are happy for both of you," I said.

The man did not speak. Ben must be asking: has he lost his speech? I said, "This is our first appointment at the speech clinic."

"Then we will not be seeing you," the woman said. "We are going to physical therapy."

Ben and I watched them as they went up the walk and through the big doors. The kinship that we felt for these two strangers helped us as we followed them up the walk to the clinic.

When we stepped into the waiting room filled with children, Ben looked at me. His eyes said: all these children. We must be in the wrong room. I was thinking the same thing.

The receptionist at the desk spoke. "May I help you?"

We walked over to her. "Mr. McBride has an appointment at ten-thirty," I said, "with the speech pathologist."

"You will not have to wait long," she told us. "Just find seats."

We took the two vacant chairs. I looked at the children: some in wheel chairs; others with leg braces or on crutches. It was evident that many had speech problems as well as the need for physical therapy.

I saw Ben smile at a red-haired boy in a wheelchair. The boy's eyes brightened as he looked at Ben's legs. Ben looked at the boy's twisted right leg and nodded encouragingly. The boy patted his leg and said, "You know what I'm going to do first? Play baseball." He went through the motion of throwing a ball and Ben pretended to catch it.

After that the waiting room was quiet; only the clicking of the braces, a dropped crutch, a smothered cough. The children did not talk. I wondered if they were afraid to trust whatever speech they had.

As I looked at Ben, it was hard to realize why we were there. I could still see him at his desk, talking with employers and applicants; dictating letters; talking on the telephone. What must he be thinking now as he sat there?

It wasn't hard to guess. He had fought his way back from other strokes; he would do it again.

Minutes ticked by. Finally the receptionist said, "You may go in now, Mr. McBride."

Ben looked at the children who had been waiting

longer than he. The receptionist explained, "Most of the children have had their therapy and are waiting for their rides home." As we left the waiting room, Ben waved to the children and they waved back.

The speech pathologist met us at the door to her office. I felt that she preferred to talk with Ben alone and said, "Shall I stay in the waiting room?"

Ben clasped my arm and shook his head. "In your case," she said, "it's all right to come in."

I found a chair on the other side of the room from her desk. Ben sat across the desk from her. I had no idea what to expect but hoped that she would ask questions that he could answer by nodding or shaking his head. She did. I was happy for him that he knew all the answers and not once did he shake his head when he should have nodded. Nor did he nod when the answer was "no." It was evident that he knew he was doing all right and was pleased.

Next, she asked him to point to certain object in the room as she named them. The picture of a dog, a horse, a train and so on. Again he did not miss but he was no longer smiling. I knew he was thinking: too easy; that's for children.

His eyes brightened when she took a box from a shelf. She picked out several skeins of yarn and placed them on her desk. She asked him to point to the colors as she named them. Again he followed through without a mistake but there was no glow of success.

When she reached for a book, he stood up and walked around to her side of the desk. "Find the word 'house,'" she told him. He pointed.

"Good. Now from the list of words to the right, pick out the words that are a part of a house." Again he pointed, and she repeated . . "door . . roof . . window. Fine."

After he had completed the exercise, I watched the pathologist turn to the back of the book. "Please, something harder," I said silently. She complied.

It was harder. Something Ben could not do. She pointed to a word and smiled encouragingly as she said, "You know what it is. Tell me."

He made several attempts before he blurted out, "Oh!"

"You are trying too hard," she told him. "Let's do it again . . . softly." He made it softer but it was still . . . "Oh." I did not learn what the word was. She said something about "Oh" being Ben's pattern. I didn't know what she meant by "pattern" and promised myself to ask later.

She laid the book aside as she said, "I am glad you are beginning therapy so soon after your stroke. The sooner we begin, the better."

Ben took his writing pad and pencil from his pocket and wrote his name for her. When she congratulated him, he wrote it again, this time with his left hand.

"You were left-handed?" she asked.

He shook his head and looked to me to explain. I said, "After he saw a man who had had a stroke and lost the use of his right hand, Ben taught himself to write with his left hand as well as with his right hand."

"And he has done all this since his stroke."

"Yes. And he has practiced until he can print several words."

Ben started to demonstrate but our half hour appointment was over. I was glad it had ended on a high note. The speech pathologist said to me, "We had a cancellation. That was the only reason we were able to see you this morning. I have no other time open this week."

I looked at Ben and thought I saw relief in his eyes. The pathologist was speaking: "Next week we can give you an appointment at nine-thirty . . . Monday, Wednesday and Friday. We make better progress when we have therapy at least three times a week."

As I started to answer I felt Ben's hand tighten on my arm. I said, "May I phone you? We do have a transportation problem."

"You don't drive?"

"No," I admitted. "But if our physician thinks Ben is ready for three trips a week, we will arrange transportation. He was released from the hospital only yesterday."

Ben was still holding my arm trying to tell me something. I knew he was worried about the therapy being too easy. If he was going to be treated like a child, did he want any more of it?

"You do have speech therapy for stroke patients," I said.

"Yes. We get a few aphasic cases," she answered.

I couldn't ask, "Are you trained to help them?" Nor could I say: I thought it was wonderful that so much was being done for the children, but since their language problems must be very different from those of the stroke victims, their therapy should be different. I said, "I will call you after I talk with our doctor."

I promised myself that before I made another appointment for Ben, I would telephone the clinic and ask about their speech therapy for adults.

While we waited for the cab to take us back to the apartment, Ben looked so dejected that I knew he had forgotten his writing success and was thinking the morning had been wasted. Nothing had been accomplished. "I don't know what we expected," I said, "Perhaps a miracle. But it doesn't work that way. It's all so new and we have so much to learn —

"Oh-oh!" he agreed and waited for me to say more.

"Maybe they have to make tests like they gave you this morning so they can evaluate —"

He shook his head and his "oh" told me it was all too childish. He would not go back until he knew he would be treated as an adult.

Finally the cab came. When the driver started to help Ben to the back seat, Ben walked around to the driver's side and started to take his seat. I knew how his hands must ache to grip the wheel again but I could only smile and say, "You wouldn't want to make the man lose his job."

The driver said, "Let me drive today. You will be driving again soon."

He would never drive again; with his loss of vision to the left in another stroke and now his lack of coordination, how was I to help him understand? When I had tried to tell him, after he lost vision to the left, that it was no longer safe for him to drive, he reminded me of a man who had lost an eye and still drove his car. Somehow he would understand.

When our cab stopped at our apartment building, I said to Ben, "I'll have lunch ready in thirty minutes." He shook his head. "I'm not hungry either," I told him. "Shall we rest a little while first?"

He was asleep in five minutes. I got out my book about aphasia. From the bibliography, I should find names of authorities on aphasia to whom I could write for information about what was being done for stroke victims.

After listing five names to write to, I read and reread lines I had underscored in the book, looking for something I could share with Ben that would help him to understand what happened to a person's brain when he lost his speech in a stroke; and what occurred with recovery.

Even with the help of the dictionary, I had difficulty simplifying the technical phrases to our understanding.

Finally I wrote, "Recovery of speech lost in a stroke depends on reintegrating the remaining undamaged brain tissues into a functioning whole."

As to what occurred in recovery: I had read that speech is controlled in right-handed persons in the left hemisphere of the brain. Ben was right-handed.

Then (this was my own reasoning) somewhere in the left hemisphere of Ben's brain, the stroke had left an injury which was the cause of his speech loss.

I wasn't sure about any of this and must check with Dr. Trippe before I tried to explain it to Ben.

Before I could read anything more, I heard Ben in the kitchenette. "Be with you in a minute," I called.

He had set the table and was writing. Sometimes he copied words from newspapers and magazines; at other times he filled pages with circles for better arm movement. Occasionally he tried a word on his own . . . just for practice. "BACIN," he wrote now.

When he showed it to me, I said, "Bacon?"

He shook his head. I was relieved. If he wanted bacon for lunch, I would have to tell him that he had had his limit for the day at breakfast. One slice, crisp and drained on a paper towel. But if not bacon, what?

Carefully he printed again . . "BACIN." I still had no idea what he meant and was afraid to guess wrong. He had had enough discouragement for one day.

Finally he drew a picture; not a very good one but I knew. "Cabin," I said.

He was so pleased that I understood, I was sorry to correct his spelling, but I felt I must. It was the only way to help him.

"Cabin," I wrote. He studied the word then copied it and looked at it again. Smiling, he circled his head with his forefinger.

I smiled with him. "You lost writing and regained it. Now it looks like we have work to do on spelling."

He circled his head again and I could no longer ignore what I knew he was trying to say . . . "Am I crazy?"

"No, Ben. Your mind is as keen as ever. You know what you want to say and you understand everything that is said to you."

I started to add: Sometimes a stroke does leave a patient so that he can't understand what is said to him (I had just read about it). That's why the speech pathologist asked you so many questions this morning. She wanted to be sure that you did understand.

This was not the time to try to explain all that. I said, "We will keep trying for speech and in the meantime keep working on writing and spelling like Dr. Trippe told us to. As well as you are writing, we'll get along."

He wrote, "EAT." I laughed. "That's telling me," and went to the refrigerator.

After lunch, he wrote, "CABIN."

"Perfect!" I said. He was still thinking about the cabin. I thought I knew why. He was thinking: Since we were leasing the farm and moving to Lawn Acres, he would not be able to finish the cabin.

"The cabin can wait," I told him, "until after we get all

the streets and utilities in at Lawn Acres."

But he wasn't thinking about the cabin; he was remembering the speech clinic. When he pointed in the direction of the clinic and shook his head, I said, "You won't have to go through that again. You feel that you wasted your time. You didn't. Instead of being unhappy, we should be happy."

He circled my head with his forefinger. I laughed. "We are happy that you came through so well." For some people who have had a stroke, the test would not have been easy.

I saw that this was hard for him to believe, and chose my words: "I have read about people who, after a stroke, have lost not only their ability to understand what is said to them, but who do not recognize people or objects. For them the test that you had would not have been easy."

He wanted to hear more so I said, "The speech pathologist cannot help the patient until he knows just how much damage the stroke has done; and what faculties are injured. You know . . . when we go to a doctor for a checkup, he makes tests; x-ray, blood tests, you know the list." He seemed convinced.

When he picked up his pencil and started to print something, I waited, hoping I would understand his spelling.

"LAND ACRE," he wrote . . then "DR. BUS." He was saying: When we move to Lawn Acres, we can take the bus into the city to speech therapy.

I agreed, "With the bus only a block from our new ranch house, we can go to therapy three times a week or as often as we need to."

"CHILFERN NO," he wrote.

"The children must have their own therapy and you

must have yours. No matter where it is, we'll find it," I promised.

I would not tell him yet about the five letters that I planned to write to the names of doctors I had taken from the book about aphasia. Surely out of the five, we would find one who could help us.

↜ 3

Living with Aphasia

The week that Dr. Trippe had asked us to stay on at the apartment in the city was over. Nancy would come in an hour to take us back to our farm home.

We were packed and waiting when the telephone rang: The speech clinic told us that the pathologist had been transferred to another city. We would be contacted when they had another pathologist.

I repeated the message to Ben and wondered what his reaction would be. His smile told me nothing. Perhaps he was glad to postpone therapy until we moved to Lawn Acres.

When he wrote, "90 DAYS," I knew he was telling me that in ninety days we would have leased the farm and moved to Lawn Acres. Then we could take the bus in to the city for speech therapy. The same clinic if they had therapy for adults; if not, we would find another.

Nancy came and we were soon on our way to the farm. When she turned off the highway into our lane, she stopped the car. She knew that we loved this view of our house under the big, old trees. The trees were bare but beautiful. Everything was beautiful.

The weather was mild for the first of March. Ben stayed outdoors so much, I was glad he seemed to know how to conserve his strength. Often, I would see him resting in the sun on the bench in our side yard.

He still had trouble using his right hand. The first time he tried to put on his right glove, I said, "Let me help."

He shook his head. It took him a half hour. Again and again he thought he had every finger in place only to find he had to start all over. He didn't want mittens. He couldn't work in them.

At last every finger was in place. He drew on his left glove and started to the barn.

There was so much for me to do, he had been gone an hour before I realized it. I looked out of the window to see if he was coming.

He was in the barnyard, looking for something. When I saw his bare right hand, I knew he had lost his glove. I wanted to help him but remembered when he put on the glove, he wanted to do it by himself.

Finally he came. When he gave me his gloves and a long cord, I knew by the twinkle in his eye that he was remembering the mittens he had worn as a child, which were connected by a cord running through his coat sleeves.

"This is the way my mother kept me from losing my mittens," I told him as I fastened one of his gloves to the cord, ran the cord through one of his coat sleeves, across the back of his coat, through the other sleeve, and attached to the other glove. It was a simple solution to a frustrating problem that brought back happy memories.

March was nearly gone. It was time that we had a lessee for the farm. Our new ranch house in Lawn Acres would not be ready before the middle of May but anyone leasing a farm would want to start an early garden. And we needed to know that we had tenants to take over when we left.

The morning I saw Ben looking at the calendar, I said, "Would you like to advertise the farm tomorrow?"

He nodded.

We wrote the ad and telephoned it to the newspaper. The first couple who answered the ad signed the lease contract.

An hour later, the doorbell rang again; another man answering our ad. I thanked him and told him we had leased the farm.

The man was going down the steps when I realized that Ben was at the door, standing in back of me. A Ben I had never seen before. When I tried to talk to him, he whirled and went through the house, pushing aside everything in his way, including me and a friend who had stopped by.

"Ben," I called after him, "I didn't know you were there. I would have explained —" He grabbed his coat and hat and was on his way to the barn before I could stop him.

When he came back he looked so dejected, my heart ached for him. Our friend had gone. I will always remember and bless her for saying, "If I couldn't talk, I'd blow my top, too."

As I looked at Ben standing in the door, I was thankful we were alone. I had had time to think and understand why he was so upset. He thought I had ignored him when he came to the door. He knew the man had seen him and that made it hurt all the more.

I remembered that the man had hesitated after I told him the farm was leased, so I said, "I'm sorry if you are disappointed." Ben would have done more. He would have shown the man the barn and around, then let me know to take his name on the possibility that we might again need a renter. I would NOT forget.

Ben was still standing at the door. "Come in," I said.

He walked over to a chair and sat down, his head in his hands. I knelt beside him. "Ben, I am sorry. You do believe me. I didn't know you were at the door." He drew me to him.

"From now on," I said, "we will answer the door together. I will explain your loss of speech but make it clear that you are still general manager around here."

He smiled and pointed to me and then to himself.

"Okay," I agreed. "We are partners."

The years that followed proved how much I needed his knowledge and experience. He needed me to understand, to think with him, and to do the talking. Whenever a business decision had to be made, whether it was in person, by letter or telephone, we went over it together until each understood every detail and agreed on what to do.

We answered the door together, and the telephone. Not until I heard his eager, "Oh!" on the extension, did I realize how much it meant to him to hear a friendly voice on the other end of the line. When in answer to his, "Oh!" there was a "Hi, Ben!" his "Oh" turned into an "Oh-oh!" that was almost a "Hal-lo-o!"

If it happened to be a business call or someone who did not know about his speech loss, I explained.

I was grateful that we had the streets and utilities to put in at Lawn Acres. It made it easier to leave the farm . . . just knowing that Lawn Acres needed us more than the farm did.

Ben had enjoyed his evenings and weekends at the

farm. Before the stroke, he always had some improvement or repair job in progress. Sometimes he worked alone. At other times he had a helper.

He had torn down the old barn and built a new one and refenced and cross fenced the entire forty acres. He had started to rebuild an old stone triple garage damaged by a tornado into a guest house to match our two bedroom bungalow. After all the hours he had spent on the garage, I wondered if he realized now that it would never be finished as a guest house.

We could still use it for picnics when we moved back to the farm from Lawn Acres. At the apartment when he wrote "CABIN," I wondered if he had written "cabin" instead of "guest house" because he couldn't spell "guest house"; or had he realized that it would never be a guest house?

After our decision to wait for speech therapy until we moved to Lawn Acres, we did nothing more about therapy. We did hear from the speech clinic but had no assurance of the adult therapy Ben needed. And we had answers to the five letters I wrote to the doctors whose names I took from my book about aphasia; all were kind but could offer no help.

We did practice writing and spelling and continued reading.

At the end of one writing session, Ben wrote, "MEN-OY." I had learned that he often transposed the letters in a word. It didn't take long to figure this one. "Money?" I said.

He nodded and looked so worried, I didn't correct his spelling. "What about money?" I asked. "We're all right."

He shook his head and wrote, "SNIRRY." I had no

idea what he meant. He wrote again ... this time, "SUNNARY."

"Summary?" I asked, trying to figure what he wanted a summary of.

He nodded and drew a line down the center of a piece of paper. Finally it dawned on me: he wanted me to list our debits and credits.

"You want a financial report," I said. "All right."

He looked so relieved, I wondered how long he had been worrying.

We made out the report together, going over each item I listed. When it was finished and I saw that he was convinced that he had nothing to worry about, I said, "Whenever you are worried about anything, let me know. Worry is not good for you; not good for any of us for that matter."

He nodded agreement. And I thought: Does he agree that worry is not good for us ... or is he promising to let me know if something bothers him? With his limited ability to communicate, how many questions does he ask himself over and over because he cannot talk about them? What courage!

As our time to move to Lawn Acres drew near, we concentrated on living to the fullest those last days at the farm. Whenever Ben wrote the name of a couple he wanted to invite to dinner, I telephoned and set the date.

I had read that some aphasic patients are sensitive about meeting people, even old friends. Not Ben.

We kept the dinners small; never more than two other couples; usually only one. Long before time for the guests to arrive, Ben started watching for them and was in the driveway to greet them before the car stopped. Everybody was so glad to see each other, that no one seemed to miss Ben's speech.

He always had his pad and pencil to carry his part in the conversation. It wasn't until the day Ruth and Paul came that I realized how little opportunity he had to use his pencil and pad.

He sat on the sofa; Paul, Ruth and I had chairs facing him. Ruth said to me, "Paul has a surprise for you and Ben."

Paul said, "You tell them."

Still looking at me, Ruth said, "We bought five registered Herefords yesterday."

"Congratulations!" I said.

Ben smiled, wrote something on his pad and offered it to Paul. Neither Paul nor Ruth saw what Ben had written. They were looking at me because I could talk. It was then that I realized people naturally direct their conversation to the person who can answer.

I went to Ben, read what he had written and gave the pad to Paul. "Polled!" he said and laughed. "Not for me. I'll take mine with pretty horns."

"HORNS," Ben wrote and pantomimed for "off." With Paul and Ruth watching, he added "BEEF" and gestured for "on."

Everybody laughed. Paul said, "I'll still take mine with horns."

From that moment on, Ben was in. He was still smiling when Ruth and Paul left. "PAUL . . CATTLE," he wrote and circled his head with his hand, telling me: When it came to cattle, Paul was crazy.

I never forgot: after that whenever we were with other people, I stayed at Ben's side.

Long after Ben slept that night, I found myself thinking about other women the world over who could not sleep because they could not relieve the suffering of their loved ones. Ben and I had much to be thankful for.

The quiet days at the farm had been good for us. We had had time to learn what Ben could do and what he could not do. He could bathe, shave and dress himself. A special rod made the bath tub safe and he liked a shower. He wore snap-on ties. He never gave up trying to do a four-in-hand but only once did he accomplish it. When he felt the occasion called for a four-in-hand, he accepted my effort, poor as it was. He managed zippers and buttons after he learned to button the sleeves of his shirt before he put it on. He usually wore loafers. He never dressed without his identification ... "I have lost my speech temporarily. Ben McBride." It included our telephone number.

Eating was no real problem. Sometimes when he couldn't manage his knife, I cut his meat. He wanted no paper napkins. They slipped off his lap, and if he spilled something, a cloth napkin was better. He cooperated on a fat and salt free diet and never forgot his medication.

Our routine was simple. We did only the necessary household and yard chores, so we could have more time to work on his writing, figuring, spelling and reading.

It took me too long to realize the extent of his reading loss. Because he understood everything I read to him, and because he had been a constant reader from childhood, and even after his stroke still read, I did not know his reading was now limited to headlines and a few paragraphs. Because I did not know that the stroke had taken his ability to concentrate on reading for any length of time, whenever he gave me something to finish reading for him, I handed it back. Wasn't that the way to help him? I had read that the patient must be encouraged to accomplish things for himself.

When he didn't try to finish whatever he had been reading, I knew something was wrong. Perhaps his glasses needed changing. His glasses were checked and were all right.

Then I read in a pamphlet about aphasia: "Often the family thinks the patient can read because he looks at a book and turns the pages when actually he does not understand what he reads. Or it may be that he understands but has lost his power to concentrate for any length of time."

Ben understood what he read; we could be thankful for that. My job was to help him until he regained his ability to concentrate for longer periods.

We practiced addition, subtraction, multiplication and division. He did well on addition, not so well with subtraction, less with multiplication and practically nothing with division.

Spelling was our biggest problem. Since so much of our communication depended on his spelling, we spent hours on it. Patiently he would write a word again and again, changing the letters, each time hopeful that he had it right.

I have forgotten what the word was that made us lose our tempers. He threw the tablet and pencil across the room.

"I've got a right to be mad, too," I said. "I am trying as hard as I can."

His look told me I was not trying. He picked up his tablet and pencil and walked out of the house. When I saw him go to the cabin and lie down on the glider on the porch, I was glad. No wonder he was tired. I was tired, too, but I could not rest until I looked in the pamphlet about aphasia to see what it said about spelling.

I read: "The aphasic who has lost spelling knows the word he is trying to write. When a person cannot figure his spelling, the aphasic thinks he is just being stubborn."

I took the pamphlet to Ben. He was asleep. I waited until he opened his eyes and smiled at me. How should I tell him? Would it upset him to be told that he knew the word he was trying to spell and thought he was spelling it correctly but he wasn't?

If I didn't tell him and he went on thinking that I was stubborn and not trying, some day he might really blow up. I decided to read it word for word from the pamphlet. When I finished, I knew we had won another victory. He was as relieved as I to understand our problem.

There was a night that really tested us. At eight-thirty, he wrote . . "HISTATISN." He wrote it over and over, changing and rearranging the letters. I tried everything I could think of. We got the dictionary and looked for words that began with "HIS" and ended with "ISN." When that failed I asked, "Is it the name of a place?"

He shook his head.

"Of a person?"

He pointed to himself. That should have been my clue but it was after ten o'clock and I was tired. At eleven o'clock, I said, "We must get our rest."

He had been in bed only five minutes when he got up and went to the living room. I followed. When he wrote, "FRU . . . ION," I said "Frustration?"

He nodded and we smiled at each other, exhausted but happy.

With all our progress, we still had our low periods when he would point to his mouth and write, "WHY?"

One Saturday night (it happened most often on Saturday nights) when he wrote, "WHY?" I surprised myself with an answer.

I switched on the floodlight in the yard and looked at the unfinished guest house . . . now the cabin. In the light, the cabin was beautiful. I called Ben to come and see it.

"Remember how the old garage looked after the tornado struck it?" I asked him.

He nodded.

"The door was blown out. All six windows gone. The roof off. There wasn't much left, was there?"

His eyes brightened. I wondered if he knew what I was going to say. "Look at it now. The old garage door is now a beautiful double window. The stones are pointed up. The new roof. The new windows. The new porch across the front . . . and your fireplace."

I saved the fireplace to the last because he was so proud of it. With a helper he had built the fireplace; inside from floor to ceiling with a heatalator. Outside on the porch was his barbeque oven with his own specially designed hickory smoke compartment. I knew he must be remembering the steaks and hamburgers we had shared with friends.

When he turned from the cabin and looked at me, I knew we were thinking together: the tornado wrecked the garage. From what we had left, we built the cabin. It was not necessary to say: "And now we have another rebuilding job to do."

‒ 4

Move to Lawn Acres

The morning of May 22, 1956, our day to move from the farm to Lawn Acres, I woke at five o'clock. Ben was not in the house. From a window, I saw him in the barnyard. Five o'clock was not early for him. Before the stroke, I once told him, "You wake the birds with your whistling." It was always some cheerful tune. "Pack Up Your Troubles in Your Old Kit Bag," and "Smile, Smile, Smile," from his World War I days, were favorites. The stroke had taken his whistling along with his speech.

As I watched him stacking creosoted posts against the barnyard fence as though he were leaving everything ready for his return, I dreaded the day before us. What would it do to him?

I need not have worried. We had planned well and Ben took pride in seeing that the movers took everything from the house except his workbench and tools in the basement. Since the stroke, he had been able to make little use of his tools. The simple act of driving a nail had become such a chore, which, once accomplished, called for a celebration. Yet every tool must be moved. They were part of him.

The work bench, the tools and the porch and yard furniture were Ben's responsibility. He had hired a neighbor with a truck to move them. By evening we were at home in our new ranch house in Lawn Acres.

The movers laid the rugs and placed the furniture. We were at home but with much still to be done before boxes were unpacked and everything was in order — all of which took time. Ben tired easily and had to rest often. Whenever he stopped to rest, he insisted that I rest, too.

We were sitting in our yard chairs when he wrote, "BUS," and pointed to his mouth. I knew he was telling me: he wanted to take the bus (only a block away now) into the city for speech therapy. How was I to tell him that I had telephoned (when he was not in the house) everywhere I could think of, trying to find a speech pathologist?

The telephone directory was no help. All it offered was the same speech correctionist that we had agreed must be for children. Not for Ben. When I saw that he was waiting for me to say something, I said, "Genevieve March's daughter may know a speech pathologist."

He didn't look very hopeful. I couldn't blame him. We hadn't seen Genevieve for years; not since her daughter was in high school. Through mutual friends we had heard that the daughter had a degree in speech and was working. They didn't know but thought it had something to do with dramatics.

Ben was still waiting. "Genevieve may know someone in speech therapy," I said. "I'll call her." I went to the telephone. When I returned he still had that not very hopeful look. I gave him the card on which I had written the name of a speech pathologist. As Ben read the name, I knew he was remembering it was the same as that of the speech correctionist in the telephone directory. "CHILD-ERN," he wrote.

"Yes," I admitted, "but he has stroke patients, too. He gives them private help." Because I had learned that it was not wise to rush him on any decision, I waited before I said, "Shall I phone for an appointment?"

He nodded. It was good to see hope again in his eyes.

We left to see the speech pathologist, happy. I was invited into his private office so I could learn how to help at home. From the beginning, it was a man-to-man relationship. No objects to name. No pictures to identify. No bits of yarn to classify as to color. The pathologist talked about things in which Ben was interested and asked him questions that he could answer with a nod or by shaking his head.

When he learned that Ben had only one vowel — "o", he tried various consonants with it. Ben had practically no consonants. Finally he managed "MOM" and "HOME." Other words were tried by sounding each letter separately . . . without success. In an effort to say "Poe," he blew out a half dozen matches trying to get the sound of "P." He got it once but was not able to do it again.

Because Ben had heard that Helen Keller's first word was "water," he let us know that if Helen Keller could say, "water," so could he. All he ever got out was "wa-." Our half hour had stretched to three-quarters of an hour. "You have others," I told the pathologist. "We must not take any more time."

While the pathologist wrote out phonetic exercises for Ben to try at home, I looked at a medical journal. When he gave Ben his lesson sheet, the pathologist said to me, "If you would like to take a magazine home, you can return it next week."

I could hardly wait to show the medical journal to Ben. It gave the case history of a doctor who had had a stroke that left him with aphasia. He misspelled "hospital" much the way Ben spelled it . . . only worse.

Once a week was all we could manage therapy. It was a long and tiring trip: our bus to the city; then another bus to the pathologist. An hour and a half each way. We practiced his assignments at home, several times a day; usually fifteen minutes at a time. When we tried longer periods, he became too tired.

Each week, I returned one medical journal and took home another. Technical as they were, I always found something that I could understand and share with Ben. At first, I had been afraid to read anything to him that might discourage him. We learned, together, that the known, however bad it may be, is better than the unknown.

When I saw the stack of notebooks the pathologist had from lectures, I volunteered to type them for him. Whatever I might learn, I thought, would well repay me. I overestimated my ability to understand the complicated, technical phrases. But the bits I did fathom made it worthwhile. And the pathologist was glad to have his notes typed.

We were eager to meet other stroke patients with aphasia. Whenever we heard of anyone who had had a stroke, Ben pointed to his mouth, asking: has he lost his speech?

We tried to contact the Smoots whom we had met at the hospital when Mr. Smoot and Ben were stroke-aphasia patients. We learned that Mr. Smoot was home. A member of the family was helping with his care. Mrs.

Smoot had gone back to her employment. Mr. Smoot's speech was returning. We were happy for them and asked them to come to see us.

It was in a downtown department store that we met Mrs. Anderton, a saleswoman. Her husband had lost his speech in a stroke four years ago. It had taken him nearly four years to regain it. They were strangers in the city and welcomed our invitation to visit us the following Sunday.

Ben and I were waiting when they stepped off the bus. Ben's eyes brightened when Rex Anderton said, "Thank you for asking us." I watched the men shake hands and wondered if Rex Anderton had had as much trouble shaking hands after his stroke as Ben had. Ben's hand-clasp had been strong and firm. After he lost his grip in his right hand, he tried to shake hands with his left hand. That was no good, so he did the best he could with his right hand.

As we started back to our house, Rex Anderton said, "I like it here," indicating our subdivision. "It's good to get away from the hotel." We knew that they lived in a small downtown hotel within walking distance of Sue Anderton's work. "We had our own home in Omaha," Mr. Anderton continued. I felt that Mrs. Anderton was encouraging him to do the talking for them but when he began to slur his words, she said: "We will buy another home some day."

Ben nodded in agreement and I said, "We hope you decide to stay here."

Before she could answer, Mr. Anderton said, "We lost everything after my stroke . . . our home, our car and our business."

"We had an automobile agency," Mrs. Anderton explained.

We had not planned to serve outdoors but when we saw how much the Andertons enjoyed the grass and trees, we set the picnic table under a tree.

While Mrs. Anderton and I were in the kitchen, taking the casserole and rolls from the oven, she said: "My husband was hired last month as a doorman at a hotel." She named a well-known hotel. "He had an accident parking a car. That was the end of his job."

"I'm sorry," I said. "It must have hurt all the more since his business was cars."

"He is still worrying about it," she said. "That's another reason we are glad to be with you today. He is so discouraged, he's afraid to look for work."

When we joined the men, Mr. Anderton was trying to figure out something that Ben had written . . . "CENTESSE COMCRETE HUMP UP PLANTER." When I saw that it was as important to Mr. Anderton as it was to Ben that he understand what Ben had written, I took the casserole and rolls back to the oven, and, all of us concentrated on solving what Ben was trying to tell us.

When he wrote "CRUB" for curb, I knew, and explained to the Andertons: "The city would not accept one of our streets here in Lawn Acres because a curb had been broken in the construction of a house. Ben is saying: if planks had been laid over the curb before the heavy trucks went over it, the concrete would not have been broken."

"The street was accepted?" Mr. Anderton asked.

Ben nodded and I said, "After the curb was repaired."

The afternoon was too short. We walked to the bus with them and promised to get together soon. We did not see them again. Mrs. Anderton telephoned that they were moving to another city.

We had looked forward to sharing experiences with the Smoots and the Andertons. Perhaps we could keep in touch by letters. We hoped that Mr. Anderton would find work within his restricted physical abilities. Perhaps in some office.

Whenever Ben put on his old farm hat and pointed to the still undeveloped corner of Lawn Acres, I knew he was going for a walk. The morning he came back, carrying his hat, I knew from the scratches on his hands and the stains on his fingers what he had in the crown of his hat. Wild blackberries! As long as the blackberries lasted, he was in the patch with his bucket every morning by five o'clock.

After the blackberries, he had another project. This included me. With a steel tape, he wanted to measure off and stake the last three lots in that undeveloped part of Lawn Acres. The fact that the surveying company, which had platted the rest of our subdivision, would remeasure and stake the lots, didn't matter. He wanted to see how close our stakes would be to their stakes. They were so close, it turned out, he couldn't slip a razor blade between them.

We practiced speech faithfully and did not miss a session with his pathologist. I marveled at Ben's patient persistence when he was making no progress in speech. He was improving in writing and spelling. Whenever I could, I set up writing exercises that he could do alone. It was good for him and gave me time to catch up with my own work.

We continued to read magazine articles; everything we could find about strokes and aphasia. Friends, far and near, sent us clippings about strokes. We wrote to every speech clinic and doctor we heard about. Their answers were kind but after reading Ben's case history, all said in effect: "We would hate to have you come here on a wild goose chase." Those were letters that were hard to show Ben, but I had no alternative. He watched for every mail.

One day when we read one such letter, for which we had watched with special hope, he became so frustrated, I didn't know what to say or do to help him.

A bulldozer was grading lots at the far corner of our tract. I could hear it. Ben always enjoyed watching any work being done in Lawn Acres, but if he heard the bulldozer now, he showed no interest. "Would you like to see how the bulldozer is doing?" I asked.

He nodded and we started out. The walk will do him good, I thought, and it's time we check on the trees. Where the woods were too dense, the locust trees were to be removed. All the rest were to be saved.

We arrived just in time to see the bulldozer bearing down on what Ben thought was an elm tree. His angry, "Oh!" stopped the operator in time. Then we saw the tree was a locust, but the operator was so furious, it took all my persuasive powers to keep him on the job.

Leasing the farm and moving to Lawn Acres, Ben had accepted. We had work to do in Lawn Acres and when it was finished, he thought we would go back to the farm. Our time in Lawn Acres was temporary.

Selling the car was not temporary. It was the first brand new, all-paid-for car we had owned; with only 12,000 miles on it. Because of his loss of vision to the left, we had no vacation drives. We often drove on little used side roads just for the thrill he had at the wheel.

After the stroke, he finally accepted the doctor's verdict that his driving days were over; but whenever I brought up the subject of my learning to drive, for one reason or another, we did nothing about it. I have wondered since, as unexpected bills had to be paid, if he realized the car would have to be sold. It was not until an unplanned-for thousand dollars in cash had to be paid on the new ranch house that he let me know his decision to sell the car.

The morning that it was parked in the drive waiting for the man who had bought it to come for it, I looked out of the window and saw Ben at the wheel. He started the motor. My first thought was, the highway is only a block away: And all the speeding cars!

"Ben," I said, trying to keep panic out of my voice, "I know what your car means to you, but —." His eyes told me I did not know. I didn't. Only a man who loved to drive, who had driven all of his adult life, could know. For him his car was *freedom*.

I could think only of the highway. He must have sensed my fear because he pointed to the dead end street with a cul-de-sac. I could almost hear him say, "Back there, I can drive."

But there were houses back there and children who played in the street. I couldn't tell him I was afraid he might run over a child.

Finally I said, "We have no right to take a chance on anything happening to the car. We don't own it any more."

He gave no sign that he heard but just sat there. He must be thinking: nothing would happen. I am still a good driver.

When he shut off the motor and got out of the car, my relief was submerged in my hurt for him. Without a backward look at the car, he went through the garage to the basement.

I returned to the kitchen and tried to wash the dishes.

Had I been wrong? Should I have gone with him and let him drive to the cul-de-sac?

He had not looked at me as he passed me on his way to the basement. Should I go to him? But what could I say? It was better for him to feel that I had failed him than to let him drive and run the risk of striking a child.

I dreaded for the new owner to come for the car . . . yet hoped he would come soon. The quicker the car was off our drive, the better.

To my great relief, Ben was equal to it. He had come up from the basement and had seen the man when he came for the car. I waited until Ben walked out to meet him before I joined them.

The new owner of the car was a neighbor. He and his wife had bought three adjoining lots in Lawn Acres, and had landscaped the ground as a play yard for their children. They had built and were living in their first house. As they could, they would build two more houses and sell them. Ben admired their foresight.

As we stood on the driveway and watched the car disappear down the street, I felt a sadness I couldn't explain. Something very real had gone out of my life . . . and I had never known the thrill of driving. What must Ben be feeling? Grounded, I thought, and wished that we could talk about it. Thankful as I was for our ability to communicate since his loss of speech, this was one time when it was not enough.

I was grateful that we had time to recover from one crisis before another was upon us. The following week we were served with a notice of a meeting of the zoning board; a petition to rezone a tract adjoining Lawn Acres on the north . . . from RESIDENTIAL to HEAVY INDUSTRY. A road machinery company wanted to buy the land. Bulldozers, caterpillar tractors, and grading machinery of all kinds would be parked alongside our subdivision.

Lots which we had sold to families who had mortgaged their future to build the house of their dreams would be worth only a fraction of what they had invested in them, if the rezoning passed.

At the meeting of the zoning board that night, the room was filled with other home owners in the neighborhood, protesting the rezoning. Too many sat in the back of the room, silent.

When Ben walked up to the long table before the members of the zoning board, I went with him and explained his loss of speech; and that he had a blueprint of our subdivision and would show them what the rezoning would do to us.

Ben spread out the blueprint. He pointed out how the entire north side of Lawn Acres adjoined the tract up for rezoning. Then with his pencil, he traced the length of our subdivision, indicated the tract that they were trying to rezone . . . and showed how it ran the entire length of our tract. To make certain that every member of the board understood, he retraced the line.

As I watched the faces of the board members, I knew he had won. "We are here not just for ourselves and the land we still own," I said, "but for all the people to whom we have sold lots and who have built homes here in Lawn Acres."

Then other people spoke for both sides. Each side had legal representation. In a few days we were notified that the rezoning petition had lost. For us, another crisis had been met and won.

For Ben, the victory was twofold. Without speech, he

had helped to save Lawn Acres. It gave him confidence to meet other crises.

I had felt his growing discouragement with his speech pathologist. He still had only two words . . . "mom" and "home." The morning after the meeting of the zoning board, he let me know that he wanted to go to the Mayo Clinic at Rochester, Minnesota. There, he would have the best in speech pathology.

I wrote for reservations.

5

To the Mayo Clinic

As the train picked up speed, I turned to Ben in the seat beside me. "It's really true. We are on our way to Mayo's," I said.

His smile told me that he was glad to hear me speak the words he had been saying to himself. "DRS," he wrote. I had learned that his "DRS" meant speech pathologists. As he pointed *up,* I knew he was telling me: at Mayo's we would have the best in speech pathology.

"I'm glad you had me write for a reservation," I told him. He took from his billfold our travelers' checks. He had written "TERLIVER BANK" as soon as we had our reservation at Mayo's. He also had in his billfold the receipt for our deposit on an apartment for a week.

It had been years since we had been on a train. The fact that the train did not go all the way to Rochester didn't bother us. Connections were good. A bus would take us the last few miles to Rochester. We would catch a cab to our apartment.

There was nothing for us to do now but relax in our comfortable chairs and enjoy from our window the changing scenes. "This is America," I said as we passed through a small town and saw a man and a small boy working in a garden. "More fun than watching television."

Ben's nod was emphatic. Next, we were passing a herd of grazing Herefords. "Oh!" he said. His eyes followed the cattle as long as they were in sight.

"Here!" I said and stood up. "You sit next to the window." Gently, he pressed me back into my seat.

It was dusk when our cab stopped in front of the beautiful, old mansion. Ben checked the address from our deposit receipt. Lucky we! For a whole week, we were to have an apartment in this dream house. As a child, I had hoped some day to live in a house with gables and windows outlined with little squares of colored glass . . . like this. As I looked at Ben now, I imagined that he had had the same dream.

The landlord answered our ring. He stood in the half-opened door. All we could see was a darkened hall and stairs that led to a second floor. "This way," he said after I told him who we were and explained Ben's loss of speech. He led us from the porch and around the house to a small stoop at the back.

Ben was still carrying our bags. I looked at him as the landlord indicated we were to follow him up a narrow staircase. Halfway up, he turned back to say, "I'd help with your bags but I have a heart condition."

I knew that Ben was thinking with me: the tiny apartment must have been servants' quarters at one time. The faded wallpaper, the dirty curtains worn to shreds and the old linoleum looked as though nothing had been done to them since there had been servants.

Ben examined the aged refrigerator and gas plate, and shook his head. I agreed; we could neither keep or eat food in this place. The landlord was showing us the shelves that he had built for our grocery supplies. "Where is the bathroom?" I asked. He opened a door to what must have been a clothes closet. "But there is no tub or shower," I said.

"You can use the tub in the bathroom in the front of the house," he said. I looked for a connecting door. There was none.

"How do we get there?" I asked; then answered my own question, "You mean we have to go down the back stairs and around to the front of the house, then up more stairs?"

Before he could answer, Ben picked up our bags and started to leave. It was nearly dark. I walked with him to the head of the stairs. "Shall we leave our bags here and start walking? We'll find another place and move tomorrow." Ben nodded agreement.

"We're sorry," I told the landlord. "You have our deposit and reservation for a week, but the inconvenience of the bathtub makes it impossible for us to stay longer than tonight. Our deposit more than pays for one night."

He was annoyed but he did not try to hold us.

Back on the street, as we started to walk, Ben pointed to another big, old house with an "Apartment for Rent" sign and shook his head. We passed several private homes with similar signs. No doubt most of them were all they should be. We didn't have time to find out. I knew what Ben was looking for: a modern apartment building.

It was dark before we found the three-story brick apartment building. It had a "No Vacancy" sign. Undaunted, Ben rang the manager's bell. She had a sublease for one week; a teacher's apartment. She would want it

September 1st. Wonderful! A week was all we needed it.

The apartment was modern, clean and roomy; a good-sized living room, bedroom and bath, and a large kitchen with a chrome-topped table and chairs. Everything spotless and shining clean!

Ben sat down at the table and counted out travelers' checks to pay our rent for the week. The apartment manager was writing our receipt when he wrote, "EAT." In our search for the apartment, we had forgotten dinner. From the twinkle in his eyes, I knew he was wishing dinner could materialize there on the table. So was I. "Where is the nearest restaurant?" I asked the apartment manager.

"There's nothing closer than eight blocks." She looked at her watch. "I don't know when it closes."

I was about to suggest that we call a cab — but if it was closed — when she added, "If you are not too hungry, there is a little grocery store —."

Ben was on his feet. "Where?" I asked.

She led us to the walk that ran the length of the apartment building. "Right down this walk into our back yard. There's a gate into the backyard of the store."

"It stays open this late?" I asked.

"The owners live in rooms back of the store. If the door is closed, ring the little bell." We were on our way.

I explained Ben's loss of speech to the elderly owners of the store.

As I watched Ben walk to the cheese and cold meats at the back, I knew that he was a boy again in another store like this one. I explained to the elderly couple, "When my husband was a boy, his father and mother had a store like yours." From that moment, the elderly couple and Ben were friends. He did all of our marketing . . . alone.

For our supper that night, we took back to the apartment a sack of bologna, cheese, crackers, bananas and milk. I couldn't remember when I had eaten bologna. I was so hungry, anything would have tasted good. As for Ben, supper was a treat.

After we had stored the leftover cheese, bologna and milk in the refrigerator and washed the dishes, Ben looked at his watch and shook his head. I guessed what he was thinking, and said, "I don't want to go back there, either. But we left our bags and told the man we would spend the night there. By the time we called a cab to bring us and the bags back here, it would be eleven o'clock. And we're to be at the Clinic by eight in the morning, remember?"

He nodded and pointed in the direction of the little store. "In the morning, you can buy what we need for breakfast," I said, "while I unpack." I should have thought of breakfast when we were at the store tonight, I told myself.

As we walked the short distance to the Clinic the next morning, I could feel Ben's excitement. Mayo's would know what to do to help him regain speech. Perhaps they would suggest some clinic. By now we knew that regaining speech could be a slow process that might take weeks. Or if they advised some new surgery, whatever it was, he would have it. He had complete confidence in Mayo's.

We had no idea that the clinic was so big, so modern and so efficient. Yet with all the routine and system, for each of us there was a special friendliness and warmth that made us forget we were strangers. It was the same for everybody: The young and the old. The rich and the poor. Men in work clothes and women in house dresses.

Executives in hand-tailored suits and women in silks and diamonds. All were the same. And as we waited for our names to be called, all were friends visiting together. We had the same hopes and the same fears. I asked a young woman at a desk how many people went through the clinic each day. "One thousand," she answered. That was in 1957. I wonder how many are seen each day now?

Ben welcomed the physical tests. He felt that he was in good condition except for his loss of speech. But it would be good to have Mayo's tell him so. And if there was something that should be corrected to help his speech, of course, he wanted to know.

He insisted that I, too, have a "physical." "Later," I promised, "after yours."

As he saw the various doctors and laboratory technicians, I was with him to answer questions that he could not answer by a nod or shaking his head. He seemed afraid to trust his writing (because of his spelling) with strangers. One time we were separated, I don't know what happened, but during an X-ray, he was taken through a door that I didn't know about. He was so upset, we did not let it happen again.

Finally the physical tests were over. We would soon have our reports. For the moment we were glad to forget them. At last, Ben was to have the test we had come for: Speech.

The speech pathologist was an attractive young woman. I liked her instantly when she greeted us in her waiting room. Since I had been invited to sit in at all of Ben's other tests, I was surprised (I hope I concealed it) when the pathologist said, "Do you mind waiting?"

"Of course not!" I said.

"Of course not," I repeated to myself as the door

closed on them. She must know, from all her experience, what is best for the patient. I could see that Ben was pleased to be on his own.

When they returned, they were smiling. Ben wrote on his tablet . . . "M.U. STEPHENES COLLEGE."

"You attended Stephens?" I asked the pathologist. Ben nodded before she could answer. I didn't know which made him happier . . . the fact that, without speech, he had been able to communicate with someone he had never seen before; or the knowledge that the pathologist had gone to Stephens years after his time at the University of Missouri . . . both in Columbia, Missouri.

The pathologist gave us no report of her testing. Eager as I was to learn about it, I understood; it took time to make a report. We were still waiting for reports on Ben's physical tests.

Our day at the clinic was over, so we went back to our apartment. Ben changed to a sports shirt and slacks, and let me know that he was going to the little grocery store. So far his purchases had been ample if not always well balanced. It was not easy to shop from day to day. At home, we planned and bought food for at least a week at a time. Perhaps just this once, I should go along. He must have read my thoughts. He handed me his notebook and pencil. "You are asking me if there is something special I want?"

I hestitated so he wouldn't guess how glad I was that he had asked, then wrote, "Lettuce .. tomatoes .. steak." I had thought of giving him a list but this was much better — for him to ask for it.

Keeping house in the little apartment took us back to our first home together. Everything was new and different. We enjoyed our walks after dinner. The grass and shrubs in Rochester were green and lush. At home the bluegrass had died and water grass had taken over.

We were glad that Ben's tests were finished. The next morning as we were getting ready to go for his reports, he let me know that I was to register for my checkup. "All right," I agreed, "as soon as we hear your reports."

"I OK," he wrote.

"I know you are," I said, thankful he couldn't read my thoughts. If there was a possibility that surgery would restore his speech, Ben would want it.

We were at the door of our apartment, on our way to the Clinic, when Ben stopped and wrote, "CUT."

I pretended I didn't know what he meant. He pointed to his lips, his neck and his head.

"Are you thinking there may be some new surgery to restore speech?" I asked.

He nodded.

"And if there is —?" He nodded before I could ask, "You want it?"

It was surgery, but not for speech. When the urologist showed us Ben's X-rays and explained (we could see without his telling us) that the kidney stones were so large that immediate surgery was a must. We walked back to our apartment in a daze. I can't remember what we had for dinner that night; or if we ate.

Ben lay on the studio couch in the living room, trying to realize what had happened to him. Only the fact that we had seen the X-rays, and our faith in Mayo's, made us accept the truth.

He pointed to his eyes (vision lost to the left) . . . to his mouth (no speech) . . . and shook his head. Surgery for speech — yes, if there was even the slightest hope of restoring it — but this . . . WHY? I was as lost as he. I didn't know the answer.

How long I sat there beside him, I have no idea. Finally, he wrote, "1 — 100?" He was asking, did he have one chance in a hundred?

"You will come through all right," I assured him. "I'm sorry I didn't ask more questions. Since you have had no pain, it can't be serious —." Or could it be? "We'll talk with the surgeon in the morning."

"1 — 100?" Ben wrote again.

"We'll ask him."

"You have a good, fifty-fifty chance," the surgeon told Ben. As he explained just what he would do, I could see Ben relax. He would enter the hospital the next morning.

We moved that evening from the apartment to the hotel across the street from the hospital.

"I like our room, don't you?" I said when the bellboy left us.

Ben didn't answer but walked to the window and looked out. Was he thinking: Emergency surgery — a strange hospital — strange nurses — a fifty-fifty chance? I didn't know what to say, so I started to unpack.

Ben closed the pullman case and led me to the door. He didn't need speech to tell me that he wanted to go down to the lobby so that we could meet some of the other guests before he left me alone.

It couldn't happen, but it did. When we stepped from the elevator, a man grabbed Ben. "Ben! What are you doing here?" he asked. In his surprise and happiness Ben seemed to forget the reason he was there. He just kept on clapping the man on the back.

I didn't know the man or his wife. Introductions could wait. We were alone no longer.

The man was H. C. Benefiel (Ben to his friends) and his wife, Ruth, from Kansas City. He and Ben were members of the Optimist Club. The Benefiels had a new car and had been patients at the Clinic long enough to know the interesting places in the area, which they promised to show us.

Since we were to be in Rochester another three weeks, Ben insisted that I start my checkup at the Clinic immediately.

"I will," I promised, "as soon as your surgery is over." I kept my promise.

His surgery was at eight the next morning. I had learned from past experience that if I saw Ben before he went to the operating room, I should be at the hospital not later than seven-thirty. I was there at seven-fifteen.

He was watching for me. We had twenty-five minutes before the cart was wheeled in for him. I followed him to the elevator and then returned to his room. Never had a room seemed so empty. I was standing at the window, looking out but seeing nothing, when I heard a suppressed sob from the room next door. Someone must be waiting in there. Alone and frightened. I went to the door.

A tall, middle-aged woman was looking out of the window. "May I come in?" I asked.

She turned. It was a moment before she could speak, "Please do." We clasped hands in silence.

Finally she said, "I got here too late. They had already taken him to the operating room. I wasn't here — and he is so very sick."

"My husband is in surgery, too," I told her. "They are in good hands. The very best. They will come through."

"But I am afraid," she said. "I know we waited too

long, but we came as soon as our doctor told us to."
Talking seemed to relieve her so I kept still and listened.
"We got here last night. We had to change planes and
that delayed us still more. This morning there wasn't
time for tests before surgery."

"Where is your home?" I asked.

"Dallas," she answered. "I know it's cancer. And I
wasn't here before he went to surgery. They told me —
eight o'clock."

I couldn't tell her; eight o'clock meant they usually
went to surgery by seven-thirty. I felt certain he had gone
before I came, or I would have heard his cart when it was
wheeled past Ben's door. "Someone will call us," I said,
"when they take our husbands to the recovery room."

Gradually we talked of other things. As I listened to
her story, told in fragments as though she must have
someone to help her bear her tribulations, I realized just
how much we do need each other. I could not think of
my own fears while she told me about their only child, a
son killed in a car accident; her own serious heart
condition; and now, if her husband did have cancer, and
they had come too late —?

At last we heard the sound of a cart in the hall, coming
from surgery. She waited at her door, and I went to mine.
I thought it was Ben's cart and stepped forward to meet
him. I couldn't see his face, only the sheet covering him
and the catheter bottle clamped to the cart. My throat
tightened as I saw the bottle filling with fluid so red, I
thought it must be pure blood.

It was not Ben. It was the man next door. "Cancer," I
heard someone say, "so advanced —." I heard no more.

Another patient was being wheeled down the hall. Ben.
His eyes told me that he was all right. His surgeon

followed and added his assurance. There was no malignancy and he had removed all the stones. I had had no fear of cancer. I wondered if Ben had been worried about it.

Mr. Harris (the patient next door) had a special nurse. Mrs. Harris left him only long enough to eat her meals. She told me later that she would not have gone out at all if Ben had not insisted that we have lunch and dinner together. I timed our being away so that I could be with Ben when his meals were served.

One morning — I don't know whether I was late or if he was served earlier than usual — I knew the moment I entered the room that something had happened. "Did you have a good breakfast?" I asked.

The expression on his face reminded me of a boy who had done something naughty and wanted to brag about it; and who, at the same time, was embarrassed and ashamed. When I didn't say anything, I imagined he enjoyed keeping me is suspense. I said nothing until he wrote, "EGG."

"Was it too soft?" I asked.

He nodded and went through the motions of pushing his plate from the tray to the floor. This had never happened before. Not that I knew of.

I started to say, "Oh, you didn't!" but changed to, "I hope you like your lunch."

Apparently, I said the right thing. His mood changed instantly. He pointed to the magazine I still held in my hand. I gave it to him. "What would you like for me to read?" I asked.

He chose an article about farming. I read words but my mind kept trying to figure out why would he gloat over throwing an egg to the floor? What had happened to him?

Not until I began research for *Silent Victory*, did I learn the answer. "Stroke patients, especially those who have lost speech, because they can no longer express themselves, will deliberately do something out of character to attract attention." "Like throwing his food on the floor," I added.

After two weeks in the hospital, Ben was discharged, but his surgeon asked him to stay another week in Rochester before his final dismissal.

We were anxious to hear the report from the speech pathologist. When we asked about it, we learned we would receive all reports, speech and physical, when we left.

From the first, Ben and I had had the same doctor in charge. It was he who gave us the final reports from our various tests. My reports were good; I was in excellent health for a woman my age. I smiled at the "for a woman my age," and started to ask, "Just what does that mean?" . . . but decided it must mean just what it said.

Ben's surgery had been successful. We were shown X-rays of his kidney minus the stones. All of his other physical tests were satisfactory.

But what about speech? I could see Ben growing tense, waiting. "And speech, doctor?" I asked.

He looked at Ben and smiled. "The stroke left you something more valuable than speech. Your keen mind."

Ben's face turned white. I had never seen him faint, but never had he received such a blow. Until this moment, we had not realized how much we had counted on Mayo's. If Mayo's couldn't help us, who could?

When I could trust my voice, I said, "Thank you, doctor. We are grateful for my husband's keen mind. You and everybody at Mayo's have been kind."

Ben shook hands with the doctor.

We had two hours until the bus would take us to the station for the train connection back home. Two hours to pay our bill at Mayo's, to go back to the hotel, pay our bill there and check out. Time enough to take care of everything before we left Rochester and Mayo's. It didn't seem possible that it was all over.

As we started down the walk from the Clinic, I wanted to turn back for one last look but was afraid of what it might do to Ben and to me. When I felt his hand on my arm, hurrying me, I wondered if he was thinking with me: it's well we have things to do before bus time; no time to think.

But I couldn't stop thinking. Why hadn't I asked the doctor to mail the speech pathologist's report to us? I would write for it.

I saw the hotel clerk give Ben the letter from our box. I knew from the expression on Ben's face he was hoping with me that it was a check for our long past due rent on the farm. We had airmailed our change of address from the apartment to the hotel to our lessees in time for them to get our check to us when it was due. The letter was from a creditor of our lessees, asking their address. That meant the farm was vacant.

On the train, going home, we pretended to read. I knew we were thinking together: we must sell our new ranch house and move back to the farm. It was too late in the season to risk releasing the farm. With so much vandalism, it must not stay vacant. We might take a loss on the ranch house, but we could not carry it through the winter. The extra expenses at Mayo's made that impossible.

When Ben dropped his magazine and closed his eyes, I

looked at him. He had dreamed of moving back to the farm. I was sorry it had to be under these circumstances. While he slept I planned the letter that I would write to the doctor at Mayo's for the report on Ben's speech. I would also write to the speech pathologist.

I never wrote either letter. I told myself I was afraid of what their report might do to Ben. Or was I fearful because so much had already happened?

It was not until I was working on the manuscript for *Silent Victory* that I wrote to Mayo's for their report on Ben's speech tests.

Their report in part: "Mr. McBride has no voluntary speech. He made use of a vowel sound for oral communication. When he attempted to imitate speech models presented by the examiner, his imitation was poor. His ability to comprehend what was said to him was quite good. By asking questions answerable by "yes" or "no," it was found that he was comprehending fairly complex material.

"In both reading and writing, Mr. McBride demonstrated considerable difference between his performance in the test situation and his performance in a more lifelike situation. Although he appeared to be severely impaired in reading in connection with aphasia test, it was apparent that he could read the newspaper and get something from what he was reading. During the test he was unable to write sentences such as 'Come in' or 'Dinner is ready', but he sometimes resorted to writing in order to communicate with Miss Simonson (the speech pathologist) and used words more complex than any he was requested to write in the test situation.

"In the area of calculation, he could handle only simple numerical concepts."

It was interesting to compare this report from the Mayo Clinic with what Ben and I had learned as we worked together for the six years we had lived with his aphasia. It encourages me to realize how much progress we made. Not in actual speech but in his ability to communicate in other ways. I can only wonder what we might have accomplished if we had had the advantage of all the research that has been done on strokes and aphasia since 1956.

This I do know, Ben would have been as grateful as I am for all the help now available to stroke victims. And if he were here, he would be helping with the writing of *Silent Victory*. Once, when we were leaving the library after another unsuccessful search for a book about stroke victims with aphasia, he wrote "BOOK" and pointed to me and then to himself.

"You want us to write a book about our experiences?" I asked. He did.

Now as I work on the manuscript of *Silent Victory* and look at the books on my shelves, all written in the last few years about strokes, aphasia and heart attacks, telling not only about speech clinics and rehabilitation centers throughout the country, but also giving easy-to-follow instructions for patients and their families who must work at home alone, I am thankful.

On my desk is a copy of a national magazine — (*Look*, June 15, 1965) I quote: "— stroke, third biggest killer, second greatest crippler in the United States." And farther on: "About 400,000 Americans will be felled this year . . . and 200,000 of them will die. Some will recover completely; others will be left in an almost vegetable condition. Most will finish their lives with residue of stroke, a limp, a useless arm, muddy speech, or aphasia, no power to speak." This in 1965.

That September day in 1957 when Ben and I left the train after our trip to the Mayo Clinic to return to our little ranch house, we faced so many problems that for the time being even speech was forgotten.

6

More Problems

As I looked at Ben across the dinner table on our first day home from the Mayo Clinic, I thought: He is so happy that we are moving back to the farm, I can't let him know how scared I am.

Before the stroke I had enjoyed the farm. He had taken the lead then. Now, without speech and with limited use of his right hand and arm, how much would he be able to do? How much could I help? How fast could I learn all I must know about farms?

While he had the employment agency, he had talked about things he would do when he could spend more time at the farm: experiment with crops and start a herd of Herefords.

What would be his frustration if I could not understand his spelling; or if I got his spelling but didn't know how to help with his project? What would it do to us?

I stopped thinking about it. He was looking at me, so I smiled and tried to make my voice sound cheerful. "We'll have all winter to make plans for spring," I said.

His answering smile told me he was already making plans. He reached for his tablet and wrote, "CATTLE."

"You want to buy cattle? How many?"

"4-5," he wrote . . . then added, "FAH."

"FAH?" I repeated, trying to figure what that had to do with cattle. When he changed it to FHA, I knew what he meant. Why hadn't I thought of it? An FHA appraisal on the ranch house in Lawn Acres would help sell it. I telephoned the Federal Housing Administration office. In a few days, we had the appraisal and loan value, and we began advertising the house.

When the first prospect came, Ben and I went to the door together. I explained his loss of speech, but that he would show them the construction of the house. He led the way to the walk-out basement, pointed out the steel beams, the steel posts and copper plumbing; then stepped off a space that could be made into a recreation room with double windows and a walk-out door to a potential patio. He pantomimed the patio and I added, "There is room for a swimming pool, too."

In spite of the fact that school had started and people with school-age children were not moving if they could help it, we had a contract on the house in three weeks. A young couple with a new baby bought it.

On November 1, 1957, we moved back to the farm. The day was dreary and slushy with falling snow. Nothing could dampen Ben's spirits. He was happier than I had seen him since his stroke.

The movers laid the rugs and placed the furniture. After they left, Ben and I walked from room to room. It was hard to realize we had been away eighteen months.

While I got supper, he laid logs in the fireplace and started a fire. I had thought we would eat in the dinette but when I saw him set up a card table before the fire, I served our plates and we carried them to the card table.

Before we started to eat, he reached for my hand and covered it with his. I could almost hear him say: "Thank you for coming back." Did he know my fear of the farm? Since his aphasia, when I couldn't figure out his spelling, I had tried to read his mind. Had he developed his own mindreading?

"I am glad to be back home," I said. His hand tightened on mine, and I wondered if he was trying to tell me that he could still manage.

At that moment a log rolled off the andirons. It took both of us to get it back. Since his stroke, he had had difficulty in placing the logs so they didn't roll.

When he looked at the books still in their packing boxes, I said, "I'll hurry with the dishes and we'll start on the books." He no longer dried the dishes for fear of dropping them.

Before the dishes were finished he had the books stacked beside their shelves and was sitting on the rug in front of the fire with his favorite book of poems. When I joined him he wanted me to read aloud. We read special passages from so many books, it was midnight before they were all back on their shelves.

That first evening back, I knew: In spite of my fear that I would not be able to help with the farm work; in spite of our lack of transportation and the possibility that we might be snowbound, we were where we belonged.

When he took a copy of Plato from a shelf, I said, "We will read everything we've wanted to read but never had time." With Plato (*Five Great Dialogs*) and Francis Bacon (*Essays and New Atlantis*) in his hand, he walked over to the end table by the sofa and placed them between the bookends. Then he turned to me and pointed to the books, telling me to choose what I wanted. I selected one about birds. We had enjoyed the birds at the farm. Now we would have time to study and really know them.

After breakfast the next morning, Ben wrote, "PAR-TUME." It was not until he led me to the north pasture fence that I knew he was trying to write "pasture." He wanted to check the pasture fences. Should he? Yesterday had been a hard day. If he rested today, tomorrow he could walk the fences. I was learning that aphasia had not changed his determination ... never to put off until tomorrow what he could do today.

When he patted his legs, I knew he was reminding me how thankful we were that he could walk. "Okay," I said, and couldn't help adding, "just the north pasture today. The others can wait." So he started off with his hammer and bucket of staples.

When he came back, he wrote "POSP WIRE FERNE WIRETENTERS STRESSER." It didn't take me long this time to figure what he wanted, but what would happen when he misspelled something I didn't know about; something not so simple as posts, wire fence and wire stretcher? I won't worry about it until it happens, I decided. All we could do was to live a day at a time.

If I worried, he would know, and worry. That, doctors agreed, he must not do. Dr. Trippe continued to see him for regular checkups and telephoned in between times. Whenever Ben wanted to do something I questioned, I waited until he was out of the house and phoned Dr. Trippe to ask if it was safe. Usually it was not only safe but good emotional and physical therapy.

It helped to learn that Ben's activities would not worsen his aphasia. Aphasia, in itself, would not kill him. But he should not overtax his heart and arteries. I knew he worried about his aphasia, so I was glad I could tell him it would not worsen. I thought of adding: Doctors agree that a person with aphasia and a heart condition can help his aphasia if he lives each day fully, within his physical ability. I decided for the present I had said enough.

Ben was careful not to overdo. When he needed help with a project, we hired a neighbor. When he tired, he sat down and rested. I hadn't realized we had so many stumps around until I saw how often he was sitting on one. If the weather was severe, he stayed inside. Doctor's orders.

Inside or outdoors, each day had its project, scheduled the night before. When he wrote, "CALBE" for cable, I knew he was going to the stream across the east pasture to see if the cable across the watergap was still tight.

As soon as he knew the fences and cable were tight, he bought cattle; not the "4-5" he had written, but a steer (for our freezer later) and seven bred cows. I was soon to learn that the responsibility for steers pastured only through the summer, as we had had them before the stroke, was entirely different from looking after cows about to become mothers.

The first cow to calve was mine; the others were ours. They all had names. Mine was Judy.

As Judy's time drew near, we shut her in the south pasture, close to the house. All during the day, we kept an eye on her; checked her the first thing in the morning and the last thing at night.

The morning I heard Judy bawling, I knew something was wrong. It was barely daybreak. I slipped out of the house without wakening Ben, and ran to the pasture. The calf, big boned and well marked, had come in the night, so close to the shallow end of the pond, his first uncertain steps must have taken him into the mire. He had fallen into the shallow water and drowned. How was I to tell Ben?

Before I could answer the question, Ben was there. He pulled the calf from the water. As we stood looking at him, Judy pressed against us. I put my arm around her neck and Ben stroked her head. Then he took her to the barn and I went for the garden cart. A neighbor helped Ben haul the calf away and bury it. After that, no expecting cow was left in the pasture with the pond.

Bessie was next to calve. We didn't know the calf had arrived until we saw it with Bessie under a tree in the meadow. It was nearly dark and looked like rain. "I'll help you get them to the barn," I told Ben. He let me know Bessie would manage.

It did rain. As soon as it was daylight the next morning, Ben and I went to the meadow. Bessie and the calf were not under the tree where we left them. She had moved her calf to higher ground. Too late, I thought, when I saw the calf stretched out as if it were dead. Bessie kept licking and nuzzling it. While Ben was feeling for its heartbeat, I went to the barn for the garden cart. When Ben saw the cart, he shook his head.

"It's not dead?" I cried.

He shook his head.

"We'll take it to the barn. It must be cold."

He pointed to the sun breaking through the clouds. I knew he was telling me that the sun and Bessie would take care of the calf. All I could see was Judy's dead calf; we could not risk losing Bessie's calf, too.

He understood. We lifted the calf into the cart and started toward the barn; Ben pulling the cart, me holding the calf in and Bessie following. We had gone less than ten feet when the calf moved a leg. Before I could tell Ben, it jumped out of the cart.

Ben didn't stop until I caught up with him. Something back of his smile made me wonder: For once, was he enjoying silence more than anything he could have said?

I didn't know what to say but finally blurted out, "Want to race Bessie and her calf to the barn?" It sounded silly; I felt silly. Slipping my hand under Ben's arm, I said, "I'm not much of a farmer. You will need patience with me." He pressed my hand between his arm and side, and I knew he was saying, "I need you."

That night when he wrote, "MEAHOW FERNE GATE," I remembered while we were in the meadow with Bessie, I had seen him looking at the old gate. So, he wanted a new gate and fence for the meadow. As our eyes met, I had the feeling he knew I understood what he wanted and that I was playing for time.

How could I say: We've already spent so much for pasture fences and gates, can't the meadow wait till spring? I couldn't say it any more than I could explain that I felt we should save the money to rebuild our emergency reserve to take care of any unexpected hospital bills.

When I couldn't hold out any longer against the eager, waiting look in his eyes, I said, "I know. You will need more hay next winter. You want to shut off the meadow so the grass will grow and you can have it cut and bailed."

He was happy that I understood, and so was I; but I wasn't prepared for what he wrote next . . . "DISK U.S. FERISHER." When I didn't get it, he tried again . . . "FERIKER."

"U.S. . . . disk," I repeated, then thinking aloud . . .

"Federal .. Fertilizer?" His "oh-oh!" told me I had it. He wanted the Federal Government program for the meadow . . . a soil test, liming, disking, fertilizing and seeding. Before I could think how to tell him our problem would be to find people with the necessary machinery to do the work, he wrote, "10' GATE DISK."

I laughed. "Okay. The gate must be ten feet wide so the disk harrow can go through it." I wasn't sure "harrow" was the right word. He was so pleased, I must have made a lucky guess.

It took a lot of telephoning; Ben helped with the directory; I did the calling. The soil test was easy. The liming and buying seed, brome, alfalfa and timothy, and having it delivered was easy. Getting the meadow disked, the fertilizer spread and the seed drilled in was the problem. Men with smaller farms who could do the work did not have the machinery for the job. Farmers who owned the needed machinery were too busy with their own hundreds of acres to do our six acre meadow.

Ben never gave up. Finally, a member of our church came to the rescue. He disked the ground, then with a combination drill and fertilizer spreader, spread the fertilizer and drilled in the seed.

When Ben handed him his check, I said, "Money cannot pay for what you have done for us; for you to take time out from your twelve hundred acres to do our small bit — ."

"I was coming this way today," he said.

"Thank you," was all I could say.

Ben clasped the man's hand and I knew he was saying, "Thank you," much better than I had.

One thing called for another. With cattle ranging over three pastures, Ben needed a riding horse. Not only to check the cattle, but he needed a horse to love. When he wrote, "HORES," I said, "I have been thinking you should have a horse," and started to add but didn't, "It must have spirit but be gentle." Why remind him of his lack of coordination? "Let's see what's advertised?" I said, and went to get our evening paper.

We found a Palomino on a nearby farm. She was so beautiful, I was happy for Ben as he swung up into the saddle and started off across the pasture. It had been so long since I had seen him on a horse, I had forgotten he was a good horseman.

When the owner of the Palomino said, "They're meant for each other," I agreed, and added, "I would love to see them in the parade next fall."

Then it happened. The Palomino whirled and started back toward the barn. Horrified, I saw Ben hit the ground — heard the owner say, "I can't imagine what happened." Then we were running to him.

When he sat up, we slowed our steps but kept going until he waved us back and started walking toward us. As we met, he held out his right hand and showed us a burn on two fingers. I knew he was using the burn as an excuse for his fall. Because of it, he had lost control of the Palomino. We agreed, glad to help him save his pride. The burn was nearly healed. I had not known about it. He had burned his hand while putting papers in the incinerator. The Palomino's owner brought salve and bandaged his hand. We did not buy the Palomino.

Ben was not discouraged. We continued to look for a horse. All we saw were either too spirited or old and worn out. Then we found the Tennessee Walker. Her official name was Independent Lady. She had been in one family all of her eight years; and was such a pet they called her Sugar.

Ben surprised an admiring audience (Sugar's owners and another prospective buyer) when he swung up into the saddle and trotted the mare off across the pasture. How could he do it — a man who had had such a serious stroke?

I wanted to be happy with him but it wasn't easy to forget how the Palomino had thrown him. I tried to conceal my fear and joined the other watchers until Ben and Sugar were out of sight. They were gone for so long, I couldn't keep from worrying.

Finally I saw them coming over a hill, taking their own time as if reluctant to return. When they stopped before us, Ben smiled and patted his pocket where he kept his billfold. I knew Sugar was his.

The days that followed were happy for Ben and Sugar. He spent hours grooming her. She had to have the best curry comb he could buy, a new blanket, halter, bridle and saddle.

Every morning she was at the pasture gate waiting for him. Later, I might look out of the window and see them galloping across the pasture so fast, I held my breath and said a prayer. At other times they were so happy, they fairly pranced, man and horse in complete rhythm.

Or, I might see them resting in the shade of a tree; Sugar standing perfectly still, Ben stretched out along her back. I couldn't tell whether he was cloud gazing or asleep.

The day they stopped to rest near the gate into the picnic yard, I joined them with lemonade for Ben and me and an apple for Sugar. "Time for refreshments," I said.

Ben sat up and smiled. He looked as though he had been asleep. He took the bridle, saddle and blanket off

Sugar, dropped them inside the gate and gave her the apple. Then we sat down at the picnic table to enjoy the lemonade.

Before he reached for his notebook and pencil, I knew he was planning a project. When he wrote, "SAW CHAIN" and pointed to a dead tree in the pasture, I said, "You want to find a man with a chain saw to saw the dead tree into firewood?"

He did; but where were we to find a man with a chain saw? The telephone directory listed only . . . "Chain Saws . . . Sales . . . Renting . . . Repairing." Then Ben remembered a friend who had had trees cut, and wrote the friend's name. I phoned him and was soon in touch with a man who had a chain saw. He would cut our tree.

As Ben returned the notebook and pencil to his pocket, I thought: Aphasia has not stopped you; only changed your course and methods. How many other men had been stopped at sixty-five, not by aphasia but by retirement? Still mentally alert and physically fit, they were bored with nothing to do.

Ben was watching me, his eyes asking my thoughts. "I was thinking about Joe," I said. Ben nodded and smiled. Joe, who had been a district credit manager, after his retirement bought a business he knew nothing about . . . a plating company.

"Joe's happy," I said. "All those beautiful old pieces he is replating in silver and gold. Learning a new business is a challenge for him."

Ben wrote the names of two other friends who had retired but were free-lancing in work they had always done; one, an accountant; the other, an engineer.

I had thought of them, too, and said, "Just because a man is sixty-five, doesn't mean he is through. He can still find work if he is willing to make adjustments."

Ben agreed.

"Would you say his best opportunity is with a small business?"

He nodded. When he smiled and wrote "EWDARDS," I knew what he was thinking.

"Yes," I agreed. "There are many retired people like the Edwards who are enjoying their freedom to travel." The Edwards had just told us about their new travel trailer and all the places they were going to see. "They have dreamed about their trip for so long," I said, "I'm glad they are on their way."

Ben's gesture said: "They can have it," as he walked over to the gate to pick up Sugar's blanket, bridle and saddle. They were too heavy to carry to the barn so he kept them in the cabin.

While he was in the cabin, I remembered how he misspelled "Edwards" and made a mental note to include it in our spelling session that evening. It worked better that way. If I corrected his spelling when he was trying to tell me something, it bothered him. By the time he rewrote the word, he lost interest in what he wanted to say.

When I saw him come out of the cabin and start toward the barn, I thought: I'll finish painting the trim on the cabin porch while he is gone. Before the stroke he was a better painter than I. But now he could no longer manage a brush.

The gleaming white paint across the front of the porch looked so beautiful when I finished it, I started on the pillars. Painting was so much fun, I forgot time until I heard Ben's angry, "Oh-oh!"

Surprised, I said, "But I thought you knew," and when

he kept shaking his head . . . "I asked you if I could paint the posts white to match the trim and I thought you nodded your head."

He grabbed the bucket, half full of paint, and threw it across the lawn. I stared in amazement when it landed straight up. Not a drop was spilled. I wanted to laugh. I looked at Ben to see if he was smiling. He wasn't.

"I did ask you," I repeated as he walked away, still shaking his head.

As I watched him go to the barn, I knew I had been wrong. I should have remembered how happy he was when he found the old railroad ties at the lumber yard. They were just what he wanted (big, strong and creosoted) to give a rustic look to the cabin. I should have known he didn't want the posts painted and shouldn't have asked . . . then I wouldn't have misunderstood him.

He was sitting outside the barn on a bench near the big, sliding door. I sat down beside him. "You have a right to be mad," I said. "I should have known better. I'm glad I didn't get any more paint on than I did. I'll take it off."

He shook his head but I could see that he was cooling off. "I'll start right now before it sets."

He shook his head again. I knew later that he was telling me . . . I couldn't get it off. I didn't. After paint remover and three coats of creosote, the white still showed through.

Ben's sixty-seventh birthday was May 6, 1958. Before the stroke, we always had a dinner on his birthday with as many as six couples. This time there would be only two other couples, long-time friends.

It was an evening to remember, sharing memories. After dinner, Ben sat on the rug before the two men on the sofa so he could be closer to them. With pencil and notepad, he kept up his part of the conversation.

As I watched everybody having a good time, I was glad that I had persuaded Ben that we should go ahead with the party and not tell anyone that I had an appointment the next day with Dr. Trippe.

The morning of May 2nd, I had awakened from a sound sleep. I don't know why I touched my upper right chest, but to my surprise I felt a small lump about the size of a navy bean. Had it come in the night? It was high enough; it should have shown above the neckline of my blouse, so I wondered why I had not seen it.

I wasn't frightened but knew I must have it checked right after Ben's birthday dinner. I would not tell him or our guests, but the day after the dinner, I would see Dr. Trippe.

That day and the next, I kept so busy I thought about myself only in flashes and gave Ben no hint of my secret. But the day before the dinner, I broke my resolution not to tell him.

I can't remember what he did that made me say, "I've got something to worry about, too." The instant the words were out, I was sorry.

He looked at me waiting for me to explain. I was so disappointed in myself, I didn't know what to say. He came to me and led me to the sofa, then sat down beside me. I told him as simply as I could.

When I finished he wrote, "DINNER," and shook his head.

"We'll go ahead with the dinner," I said. "Look!" and I showed him how small the lump was. "It's probably nothing at all but I will have it checked the day after the dinner, I promise."

When I finally persuaded him not to call off the party, I said, "Let's get the table ready now, then it will be done for tomorrow."

We had combined our dining room and living room. Our only piece of dining room furniture was the drop leaf table that we opened out when we had more than two guests; at other times we ate in the dinette.

He didn't move until I started toward the table. We set it and no more was said about my seeing the doctor until the morning after the dinner.

I was thankful we had our appointment. In five days the lump had nearly doubled in size and was burning and stinging. Still I could not think it was anything serious.

"I don't think it amounts to anything," Dr. Trippe said, but he telephoned our surgeon and sent us to him on our way home.

The surgeon said, "I don't think it is anything to worry about but meet me at Research Emergency tomorrow morning at ten and we'll do a biopsy."

Nancy (our daughter) took us in for the biopsy. It was made and we went home to wait for the report from the laboratory. I still was not worried: the biopsy was only to give assurance, I told myself.

Two days later when the telephone rang and I heard the voice of the surgeon, I thought: How good of you to take your time to call when your nurse could have phoned. "I'm sorry," he said, "We'll have to put you in the hospital."

It was a long moment before the full impact of his words hit me. As soon as I could trust my voice, I said, "When?"

"Today. I want you there by four this afternoon."

"We'll be there," I promised.

Ben was at the cabin. I ran out of the house, crying. He met me halfway up the path. "It is cancer," I sobbed. Never had his arms been so gentle and strong. I remember thinking: His arms are strong but he drops things.

As I felt his heart beating against mine, I stopped crying. "I'm not afraid now," I told him. "I have to check in at the hospital by four. Nancy will take us."

7

Another Speech Clinic –
Aphasic Friends

The next morning my brother Ray, his wife Ruth, my sister Ellamae, and Nancy were to wait with Ben while I was in surgery.

As my cart was rolled out of my room, and I knew I was on my way to surgery, I had a strange, detached feeling until I heard the voice of the anesthetist; then, as I drifted away, I was conscious of my unspoken words . . . I am not afraid — not a-f-r-a-i-d.

Later, when I was back in my room with the same around-the-clock nurses Ben had, I felt no pain, but my right chest and arm were heavy with bandages. I saw nothing, for my eyes were closed; heard nothing, except my own words, "I want my husband."

"He is right here," Ellamae said.

I opened my eyes and there he was, smiling down at me. As his hand closed over my free left hand, his strength was mine. Still smiling, he tapped the back of my hand with his forefinger . . . one-two-three. And I answered . . . one-two-three. "I love you" . . . our secret code since early courtship days.

The next morning I woke before daylight, gripped by

an overpowering fear. What if they hadn't found all the cancer? What if—? I couldn't face it. "I can't leave Ben," I thought as I smothered the sob in my pillow.

My assurance came as clearly as spoken words . . . *As long as Ben needs you, you will be here.* Calmed, I went back to sleep. I never lost faith again.

The next day the nurse said, "You will be ready to start therapy tomorrow," "Therapy?" I asked. Would I have therapy like a stroke patient?

She smiled, "You might try to raise your arm today."

"Watch!" I told her as I lifted my right arm. She was surprised and pleased.

Ben stayed home alone the two weeks I was in the hospital. Nancy brought him to see me every day. She told me afterwards that every morning when she went for him, he had finished his breakfast, washed the dishes and was ready and waiting for her.

Usually he wore a sports shirt that he could button, a slip cord tie and loafers. He declined all dinner invitations except one with Nancy and her family the day of my surgery. He wanted to be home near the telephone. He wanted to be HOME.

We made arrangements for me to have twenty-two X-ray treatments, three a week, immediately after my release from the hospital; also, I would have regular checkups by a radiologist indefinitely.

Until the treatments were finished Ben and I did little but rest. The trips into the city were tiring.

On one trip we stopped at our lawyer's office and learned that he had a client who was living with aphasia. Gene McCoy's stroke followed by aphasia occurred in April after Ben's stroke in January 1956. As soon as I finished treatments, we invited the McCoys to dinner.

Before they came we met the Humphreys. Bill Humphrey had suffered a stroke in 1953 that left him with aphasia. We invited the Humphreys to join the McCoys at our home.

Gene's "ei" and Bill's "yeh" and Ben's "oh" established an immediate bond. With broad smiles and pats on one another's shoulders (Gene and Bill were left-handed because their right hands were useless), the men made their way to the cabin porch; Ben in step with Gene and Bill, each of whom walked with a cane and a fitted shoe brace on the right foot. Delpha McCoy, Marie Humphrey and I followed.

As we joined the men, we saw that Gene was showing Bill and Ben his new shoe brace. Bill motioned for Marie to examine it. "It is lighter and more comfortable than yours," she told him. "We'll buy you one like it."

"Yeh, yeh!" Bill agreed.

"Bill and I are selling greeting cards," Marie told us. "He loves getting out and meeting people." Bill nodded and smiled.

"When Gene tried to tell Delpha something and couldn't make her understand, Ben offered him his tablet and pencil. Gene shook his head. We learned later that Gene and Bill had only limited writing. Finally, Gene made a circle with his thumb and forefinger and raised it to his mouth.

"Apple," Delpha said.

Gene nodded and smiled.

"He wants me to tell you about the apples we brought back from the farm last week," Delpha explained.

Gene nodded and pointed to Bill and Ben.

"We want to share the apples with you," Delpha agreed. "They make good pies and sauce."

After we thanked them, Marie asked, "How far is your farm?"

"A two hour drive," Delpha said. "We rent the land and keep the house furnished so we can stay overnight or as long as we like. We used to stay a week or two at a time but Gene's boarder stopped that."

"Gene's boarder?"

Gene nodded and beamed as Delpha explained, "We rented our guest room to a young man who teaches in our high school. When he asked about breakfast, Gene let me know he would take care of breakfast for him."

"And he does?" Marie asked for the rest of us.

"Indeed he does," Delpha said. "Fruit, cereal, bacon to a crisp and eggs done to the second."

As we applauded, I thought: Gene, before his stroke, was a salesman for a national electrical company; Bill was a farmer, businessman and mayor of Weston, Mo. before his stroke; and Ben . . . each making his own adjustment and happy.

When Ben looked at me and pointed to his mouth, I knew he couldn't mean dinner (it wasn't time yet), but what —? Then he pointed to Bill's mouth and to Gene's mouth. Speech, of course.

"Ben wants to know if Bill and Gene have had speech therapy?"

When Delpha said, "Gene has had therapy," Ben signaled for me to get the name of the pathologist.

Later when Delpha, Marie and I were alone in the house, Marie said, "Bill's doctor told me that therapy would not help Bill regain speech."

"Speech therapy has not helped Gene," Delpha said. "But we will continue as long as he wants it."

"Have you found any books about aphasia?" I asked.

They hadn't. "With all the progress that is being made in the medical world, we can hope for help before long," I added.

"I am glad Gene enjoys taking walks in the neighborhood," Delpha said. "He goes alone and likes to meet people."

"Bill likes to meet people, too," Marie said. "We often go out to dinner. He can say, 'Yes' and 'No' and some words, but he knows he does not pronounce them correctly so says them only to me unless I ask him to say them for someone. He practices copying words and can sign his name but he does best in arithmetic. He now adds ten numbers across and ten down and gets the correct answer."

"Gene likes to have company," Delpha said. "We want you to come to our house."

"Bill and I want you, too."

"And you must come back here, I said. "It's good for the men to be together — and for us."

After dinner we agreed that we would meet next time at the Humphreys, then with the McCoys and back to us.

The McCoys lived to the south of us, the Humphreys to the north. Delpha said to Ben, "When we go to the Humphreys, we'll stop by for you," and Marie added, "Bill and I will pick you up when we go to the McCoys."

Ben looked at me and held up two fingers. I knew we were thinking together and said, "Ben and I want you to come here twice for each time we go to your house."

As I looked at Delpha and Marie, I told myself I would learn to drive as soon as possible.

The next morning, Ben had me telephone Gene's pathologist for an appointment.

Now that he understood the importance of evaluation

tests, Ben went through the speech pathologist's examination with a smile. At the end of the first lesson, he was still smiling; but after five lessons with no progress, I asked myself how much longer he could continue?

He answered the question on our way home. As we left the pathologist, he tapped his mouth and shook his head. He looked so discouraged, I said, "We won't go back if you don't want to." When we reached home, he pointed to the telephone. "You want me to call the pathologist now?" I asked.

He nodded. I would have preferred that he had not been listening when I phoned. When the pathologist answered, I said simply, "Ben feels that he is not making any progress and wants to discontinue therapy."

I was glad he did not hear her answer, "I am sorry," she said, "that I have not been able to help him. Some patients need therapy to keep up their courage. If they feel we are trying to help them, they don't lose heart."

While I was trying to think how to answer, Ben touched my arm and showed me his billfold. I said, "Ben wants me to ask you if we have paid all we owe?" I knew we had because I wrote a check for each lesson when it was over.

After that was settled, I hoped Ben would feel better. He was still unhappy. I walked to the window and looked out. "It's too nice to stay inside," I said. "Let's go to the cabin."

He did not answer but sat on the sofa, his face expressionless. I started to go to him, then decided he wanted to be alone. "I'm going to the garden," I told him. "The tomatoes haven't been picked for two days." Perhaps he would come, too. He didn't.

He was still on the sofa when I returned, staring at something he had written . . . the name of a friend, who, the first time he saw Ben after his loss of speech, had called him "Dummy". Before the stroke, they had kidded each other. He must have forgotten that Ben could no longer talk back. Or perhaps he was embarrassed and was trying to be funny. I knew he would not have hurt Ben intentionally. Other people had worried about what to say.

One of Ben's best friends said to me after the stroke, "I'm afraid to see Ben. I don't know what it will do to him . . . and to me." When they finally met, they were so happy to see each other, they didn't need speech.

When Ben again wrote the name of the man who had called him "Dummy," I knew I had to do something. I had learned that the best way to help him out of his dejection, was to remind him of something happy. But the timing had to be right. He couldn't be rushed into it.

So I picked up a book of house plans and started to look through it. Sometimes that worked. He spent hours studying house plans, but he wasn't interested now.

Finally I said, "When Nancy comes tomorrow, shall we ask her to take us to Lawn Acres? I would like to see the new house on Lot 23. Wouldn't you?"

He didn't answer but he closed the tablet and laid it aside.

"If anyone had told us a year ago when we moved back to the farm, that all of the lots on both sides of 77th Street would have been sold and houses built by now, would you have believed it?"

His smile told me that I could now say what I had been leading up to: "Remember what Betty (another friend) said when we showed Lawn Acres to her?"

He nodded and I repeated Betty's words, "Ben, when did you learn the real estate business? You certainly were foresighted to buy all this land."

His "oh-oh!" said how well he remembered and how happy it made him.

A few minutes later he gave me a magazine and pointed to an editorial he wanted me to read aloud. When I finished, he wrote, "LETTER."

"You want to write a letter to the author?" I asked. We had written other authors about their articles and books but this man was the publisher of one of our biggest national magazines.

Ben nodded and started to underscore the lines in the editorial that he liked best. So I drafted the letter. We went over it together; I typed it, and Ben signed it.

A week later, I could hardly believe my own eyes when Ben handed me a letter from the magazine: "This is to tell you how much I appreciate your letter of July 24th, . . . Your encouraging words about this feature mean very much to me." It was signed by the publisher of the magazine and author of the editorial.

While we were basking in our happy surprise, more mail came; a copy of the magazine publisher's latest book autographed . . . "For Ben McBride . . . with best wishes from . . .", again the signature of the magazine publisher.

That started us on an extensive reading program . . . magazines and books. Television was almost forgotten. We always had been selective in choosing television and radio programs because we preferred to spend our time reading.

Until now, reading had been for pleasure and interest. It meant much more to us when we started to think with the authors. We wrote letters to them, telling what we liked and what we didn't.

We also wrote famous people about the opinions they

expressed in newspapers. And after we realized the power of television, we watched more programs; and wrote to the networks, telling them which programs (with the station, name and date) we wanted to see more of, and which ones we could do without. Always we told our reasons. Ben signed each letter. Not once did we mention his aphasia.

Some of our letters were not answered but the response from publishers, editors and the networks in general convinced us that they desire to give us their best and appreciate our telling them what we want.

One magazine editor wrote, "I can't tell you how much we appreciated your nice letter about —, appearing in our June issue . . . It was very good of you to take time to write to us."

After his stroke, Ben continued to go to his barber friend in the city for his haircuts. It worked out well. When he needed a haircut, we made a day of it; lunch downtown, shopping and errands.

We had been so busy writing to publishers, editors and networks, he was long overdue for a haircut. The morning he looked in the mirror and ran his fingers through his hair, I said half joking, "I'll cut it for you."

He looked so skeptical, I determined to show him I could do it. "Remember the clippers we bought and never used?" The idea had been that I might trim around the edges of his hair sometimes and save a trip to the barber. I had never had the courage to attempt a neckline trim, and here I was, offering to do a haircut.

When he still looked doubtful, I said, "If you want me to phone for an appointment for you —?"

He grinned and patted his billfold.

"It doesn't make sense," I agreed, "to pay cab fare to

the city just for a haircut."

So I brought out the clippers. I knew he was thinking, what about scissors and a comb? So was I. We found a comb that would do, but my scissors were a poor substitute for barber shears.

With makeshift equipment and no experience, what kind of a job would I do? I had never watched the barber cut Ben's hair. That had been my time to hurry and get done the errands I knew would tire him.

I tried to remember what little I knew about how barbers worked. First, they fastened some kind of a band around the neck. What could I use for a band? Ben found the answer by folding one of his handkerchiefs and showing me how to pin it around his neck. While I was trying to think what to use for that sheet-like deal that would cover him from the neck down, he gave me our biggest bath towel. Another poor substitute, but the best we had.

Everything ready, Ben pointed to the bench in our side yard. "Fine," I agreed. "No hair on the floor to vacuum," and to myself added: we'll need all the fresh air we can get.

When he saw me looking at the clippers, he rubbed the sides at the back of his neck. But did I use them before or after the haircut? Might as well start with them, I decided. Thank goodness they are not electric. I'd scalp him for sure.

I finished with the clippers and Ben handed me the comb and scissors. Which side first? I started on the left, moving the comb slowly and clipping the hair that showed between the teeth. Not too difficult. The trick would be to keep it even all the way around.

The left side finished, I started on the right. I felt Ben

become tense when the scissors touched his ear. "I won't nick it," I promised. The sides done, I walked around to the front to see how they looked. They matched better than I had hoped for. Ben grinned and patted the thinning hair on top of his head.

"I won't touch it," I promised. "Do barbers charge less for doing only three-fourths of your head or do I skip the tip?"

He grinned and offered me a tip.

When he lowered his chin so I could start on the back of his head, I sighed with relief. I was almost done. But the back of his head took as long as the sides. I couldn't make it match the rest. Finally, I had done the best I could. Then I saw hair on his neck where I thought I had clipped it. I must have missed that spot. Hair couldn't grow that fast.

And there was an uneven spot in the center back where I had used the comb and scissors. Perhaps I could touch it up with the clippers. Before I realized it, there was a strip up the back of his head, nearly bald. And I had thought I was giving it a light touch. What would he say? How long would it take for the hair to grow out? If he ran his hand over his head, he would feel it. Or, suppose he looked in a mirror with a hand glass?

He did neither. As we passed the mirror in the hall, he paused, turned his head from side to side, and nodded his approval. I never knew whether or not he learned that I had nearly scalped him, but the next time he needed a haircut, I said, "Shall I phone for an appointment for you?" I was prepared to insist if he had said, "No."

His "oh-oh!" for "yes" was so emphatic, I telephoned at once.

The day that Ben gave me the magazine with the article

about the Institute of Logopedics at Wichita, Kansas, I knew he had found a new hope for speech.

We wrote to the Institute. Their report on the help they had given to victims of stroke and aphasia was sufficiently encouraging to induce us to plan to go to Wichita.

Such a wonderful speech clinic, why hadn't we heard about it before? If, after his evaluation test, Ben was accepted, we would rent a little apartment near the Institute and stay as long as it took for him to regain speech.

Before we could complete arrangements to close the house and go to Wichita, we had warnings that Ben's heart condition had worsened. Even to regain speech, we could not leave his doctor and hospital. Another disappointment. How would he accept it?

I couldn't tell what he was thinking. He was quieter and rested more. Good for his heart. But he had not given up hope of speech therapy, that I knew, even before he brought me the telephone directory and pointed to "Institute of Logopedics" and the telephone number.

"They have a speech clinic listed here," I said.

He nodded and pointed again to the telephone number.

"I'll call right now."

The Clinic was a part of the Institute of Logopedics at Wichita. How wonderful! We couldn't go to Wichita but one of their speech pathologists would come to us. It was settled when I explained our transportation problem. The speech pathologist arranged to come to our home in the evening after his day classes.

Undoubtedly, Ben would have made better progress if he could have had the intensive training at the Institute in Wichita, but we were thankful the pathologist could come to us once a week. After each lesson he left enough homework to make it equal to two lessons a week.

At our first meeting, the speech pathologist told us, "In fairness to the patient, if after eight or nine lessons there is no improvement, therapy will be discontinued."

"That is the way it should be," I said, and Ben nodded in agreement. I knew from the expression on his face that he was thinking: At last I have found the man who will help me regain speech.

As I looked into his eyes bright with hope, I thought: Thank God for hope and faith.

8

Try Hypnotism?

No man could have been more dedicated to his work than the speech pathologist from the Institute of Logopedics; no patient could have tried harder than Ben. He tried too hard. Even his "ohs" were strained and unnatural.

The only way Ben knew how to accomplish anything was by willpower and hard work.

At the end of nine weeks, he still had no more than "mom" and "home," the two words he had regained after the stroke.

When the speech pathologist and we agreed to discontinue therapy, Ben wrote, "IMPOSSILLIP." He was trying to say, "It doesn't seem possible."

What could I say or do to help him? What hope could I give him? I groped for something to restore his courage. If only he could talk (I knew by the expression in his eyes there was much he wanted to say), we could work it out together.

Finally, I said, "Remember that last letter that you and Jo Melcher (his secretary) did together?" It was another try at bringing back happy memories. I had learned that recalling some accomplishment of his, or a word of praise, helped to break the spell of his dejection.

For a moment I thought he hadn't heard me. When I saw the flickering of a smile, I said, "Remember how you both laughed when you finished dictating?"

He nodded.

"You never had been able to dictate too fast for Jo to get it. Remember that time you thought you had won?" I could see that he was remembering. "But you hadn't. She had every word."

He smiled and wrote, "2."

"Yes, it was two pages and a very important letter."

He nodded.

"And you were as happy as Jo was that again she had won. You know what she said to me later?" (I knew he remembered but he needed to hear it again). "Quote . . . 'I have taken dictation from a famous commentator and top executives but to my way of thinking, Ben McBride has the best command of the English language of any of them. His sentence structure is perfect.'"

His smile faded. He must be thinking: And now I can't speak or write a simple sentence.

I had said too much. I should have stopped while he was still smiling at the memory of the letter. What could I say now?

He wrote, "CHRUCH." I didn't know why he wrote "church," but I was glad that he was thinking about something else.

"You want to go to church next Sunday?"

He shook his head. I should not have asked the question. After the stroke, we had gone to church only two times. When the singing started, he couldn't keep the tears from running down his cheeks. I wondered now if I should have told him that I had read that stroke victims sometimes cried.

He had let me know that he wanted to stay home and listen to the church services on TV and radio, so I had thought no more about going to church.

But why had he written, "church?" While I was trying to think what to say, he wrote, "RIGGED CROSS OLD THE."

I remembered the last time we went to church, they sang, "The Old Rugged Cross." It had been a favorite of his; as it had been of his father and mother.

When I saw that he was waiting for me to say something, I said, "The next time the Curtis Dotsons (Mr. Dotson was a soloist at our church) come, would you like for him to sing, 'The Old Rugged Cross'?"

Before I finished the question he nodded. "I would like that, too," I said.

He was smiling when he went to the barn. Once again we had won a bout with despondency.

The Dotsons often came to see us but never went near our organ. I knew why . . . they had seen Ben's tears at church when the singing began.

When I telephoned Mrs. Dotson and told her that Ben would like for them to sing the next time they came, she said, "We'll see you next Sunday."

Our organ was the old-fashioned treadle kind. I was happy when we found it in our neighborhood, refinished and in perfect condition.

When the Dotsons arrived, Ben met them and led them to the organ. As soon as Mrs. Dotson was ready to play, he placed a hymnal before her, opened to "The Old Rugged Cross."

I stood back, thinking Mr. Dotson would sing a solo.

He barely started when Ben's "oh-oh" joined in. By the time they reached the chorus, Mrs. Dotson and I were singing, too. We sang all four verses . . . Ben's off-key "oh-oh" loudest of all.

He didn't seem to realize that he was off-key. He was nearer speech than he had been since the stroke. I can still see him standing there, face uplifted, pouring out his heart in song.

As soon as we finished "The Old Rugged Cross," he had another hymn for us to sing . . . and another and another for an hour. As the Dotsons were leaving, I said, "You have given us such a happy afternoon, I don't know how to thank you."

"We've enjoyed it, too," Mr. Dotson said, and his wife added, "It has been a happy time for all of us."

Ben clasped their hands, and they knew how much it meant to him.

The next day Ben had some project (I have forgotten what it was) but he needed certain sized screws.

He wrote, "SERWS . . HDW."

"You want to go to a hardware store and buy screws?" I asked.

He nodded.

We enjoyed our trips to the city. At our bank everybody, from the custodian to the president, was Ben's friend. On the streets he met people whose, "Hi Ben!" brightened his whole day.

Shopping sometimes was a problem. Because it was hard to make salespeople understand what he wanted, I tried to learn ahead of time about what he might want so I could help. And after he bought a pair of shoes that were twice the price he thought they were, I learned to make sure that he read the price tag.

Most of our hardware needs we bought in a small store not far from home. The owner helped Ben find whatever he wanted. Once, when it wasn't convenient for us to go to the store, I telephoned Ben's order and asked the storekeeper if he would mail it to us.

He said, "I'm coming your way tonight and will bring it."

This time, since we had no way of getting to the store closer home and to the bank, we took a cab to the city. That meant a big hardware store, but Ben had shopped there before and always had been able to make the salesmen know what he wanted. This time he had a new salesman.

Too late I realized that I should have learned what kind of a screw and size Ben wanted. Always before, the salesman had pulled out different drawers of screws and Ben had pointed to the ones he needed.

When at last he found the kind of screw he thought he could use, he couldn't make the salesman understand the size he desired. He wrote, "3/8 — 5/8."

I repeated, "3/8 . . . 5/8."

Ben shook his head and again wrote what looked to the salesman and me like "3/8 . . 5/8." I wondered later if he was trying to tell us that he wanted a size between 3/8 and 5/8?

When Ben kept writing "3/8 . . 5/8", the salesman closed the drawer. Ben whirled and walked out of the store.

I followed . . . just in time to see him step from the sidewalk into the street. The light had just changed and the oncoming cars were almost on him when I jerked him back to the sidewalk.

I could feel my hand trembling as I held on to his arm.

Not suicide. He wouldn't try. He had had more frustration than he could take and was running away.

I must find a telephone and call a cab to take us home. As we walked away, I saw the salesman watching us from the door of the hardware store. I hoped he knew everything was under control.

We always called the small cab company that catered especially to north-of-the-river patrons. The drivers were our friends. They realized how much Ben missed driving his own car and pointed out anything new along the highway. They told him about new developments and kept him informed on the progress of new highways.

I was grateful when we were safe in the cab and on our way home. Ben greeted the driver then sat back and closed his eyes. The driver looked at Ben and turned to me.

"He is tired," I said.

"Ben," the driver said, "I am going to take you home over the new highway."

Ben's "oh-oh!" made me think he was trying to say, "But it is out of your way."

"It's out of your way," I said. "Can you spare the time?"

"It's about the same distance. It won't take any longer."

Ben's "oh-oh!" told us how much he wanted to see the new highway.

"Thank you. We will enjoy it," I said.

The driver's kindness and the ride helped Ben forget the hardware store. By the time we reached home, he was smiling.

When the cab stopped at our house, he pointed to a tree of ripe peaches. He brought a basket and let the driver know that he wanted to share the peaches with him. Together they filled the basket.

I never learned what kind of a screw or the size Ben wanted. I was glad he did no more about it.

The day he took an encyclopedia from the bookcase and called his "oh-oh" for me to come, I turned off the electricity under the green beans I was cooking. I thought he had something he wanted me to read.

He opened the book, pointed to "BYRON, GEORGE GORDON BYRON, 6th BARON (1788-1824)" and gave it to me. When I started to read, he motioned for me to stop and close the book.

So I wasn't to read, after all. It wasn't anything that he had been reading. He had just come in from the barn. Probably something he had been thinking about while he was at the barn. It was . . . I knew when he limped across the room.

"Lord Byron was lame," I said.

Ben nodded.

"I had forgotten until you reminded me." He was pleased that we were thinking together. Then by pantomime he let me know that Lord Byron could swim and that he played cricket.

I must have looked vague, trying to remember; Ben motioned for me to open the encyclopedia. I read . . . "He was a 'record swimmer', and in spite of his lameness, enough of a cricketer to play for his school at Lord's."

I smiled at Ben. "Your memory amazes me. I don't know when I've thought about Lord Byron." He pointed toward the barn, confirming what I had surmised. "You were thinking about him while you were at the barn?" I asked.

He nodded and patted me on the head as if I was smart to guess. "I wish I could remember history the way you do," I told him, and thought: Praise spurs each of us to do our best. How much more it means to someone with aphasia!

I kept thinking about it; marveling at Ben's storehouse of knowledge, and how often he drew on it when he was alone; as when he was at the barn and thought about Lord Byron. But why Lord Byron? Was it because Lord Byron had not let his handicap stop him? Did Ben renew his courage by remembering the courage of others?

After dinner that night when Ben started to write in his notebook, I knew from the expression on his face that it was something special. I glanced at the clock. Fifteen minutes later he gave me his notebook. From memory he had written the names of thirty-two of the thirty-four presidents of the United States in perfect order, with one exception; he transposed James Madison and James Monroe. Twelve he had spelled correctly and many others were easy to figure out ... "H. Q. ADAM" for John Quincy Adams ... "TYRIL" for Tyler ... and "PLOK" for Polk ... as examples.

Again, I was amazed at his memory and the fact that his spelling was better than usual when writing the names of the presidents.

It confirmed what I read later in *Time,* May 11, 1962: "The technical name, aphasia, covers far more than its literal meaning, loss of speech. Usually neither innate intelligence nor accumulated knowledge is destroyed, but access to each is cut off from the patient by a breakdown in his communications system. The breakdown may damage the receptive (reading and listening) functions, or the expressive (speaking, gesturing, writing), or both in infinitely various combinations."

Ben was so pleased with his success in writing the names of the presidents, he motioned for me to come and sit beside him on the sofa while he wrote something else . . . "GLDLASTOME PURCHURSE 1849 . . AZIS-TANO . . PIESE NEWICE." Now, what was he trying to tell me?"PURCHURSE" must be Purchase . . . 1849? What happened in 1849? Was "AZISTANO" Arizona? And "GLDLASTOME" . . . not Gladstone . . . maybe "Gadsden?" I asked.

He nodded and again patted my head. So we turned to the encyclopedia and I read, "GADSDEN, JAMES (1788-1858). In 1853 President Franklin Pierce appointed him (Gadsden) minister to Mexico, with which country he negotiated the so-called 'Gadsden Treaty' (signed December 30, 1853 — Ben's 1849 was close) . . . and provided for a readjustment of the boundary established by the treaty of Guadalupe Hidalgo, the United States acquiring 45,535 sq. mi. of land, since known as the 'Gadsden Purchase' in what is now New Mexico and Arizona."

When Ben returned the encyclopedia to the bookcase, he pointed to the clock. We had lost track of time. It didn't matter that it was midnight. It had been worth losing a little sleep.

Happy days followed until the morning he looked at me across the breakfast table. I knew from the expression in his eyes that something was wrong.

When he wrote "DREAN" and pointed to his mouth, I knew that he must have dreamed that he had regained speech. It had happened before and always left him depressed.

I could imagine what he went through . . . to hear

himself talking — to awake and try to speak — only to
find that he was still without speech. I tried to think what
to say.

Did he sometimes have dreams that were happy
memories? Or did he ever dream about himself in a
situation so terrible, it was a relief to awake and find it
wasn't true? That sometimes happened to me, but I
couldn't tell him now. Again, if we could just talk things
over as we used to, how different life would be for both of
us.

After breakfast, he stood at the window looking out
while I did the dishes. His "Oh-oh!" took me to the
window. A car had turned into our driveway. "Welcome!"
I said to myself, "whoever you are."

It was a friend who had just been to a meeting of her
club. She was still excited about the amateur hypnotist
who had been on the program. I don't think she realized
what ideas she might give Ben but when I saw the way he
was taking in her every word, I knew the damage had
been done. He was thinking: Perhaps hypnotism is the
answer. If it can bring back my speech—?

I felt that hypnotism in the hands of an expert could be
valuable in medicine, psychiatry and surgery. But this
man was an amateur. For Ben he could be dangerous. If
Ben wasn't so desperate for speech, he would agree.

I said nothing until our friend left and then waited for
Ben to make the first move. I didn't wait long. He
opened his notebook to the name and address of the
hypnotist. He had let our friend know that he wanted it
and she had written it for him.

While I was still trying to think what to say, Ben
pointed to the telephone.

"Don't you think that a letter would be better than a

telephone call?" I suggested. "In a letter we can give the facts about the treatment you have had so far. It would help him to have the history of your aphasia." I could see he was thinking, and added, "Whenever we write to a new doctor or speech clinic, we always give your history."

Finally, he nodded in agreement. We drafted the letter, I typed it, and Ben took it to our mailbox on the highway.

9

Heart Condition Worsens

Because the address of the hypnotist was local (our little farm had recently been annexed by the city), Ben started looking for an answer two days after he mailed our letter.

I still didn't know how I was going to handle the situation if the hypnotist said he could help Ben. I had checked on him, telephoning while Ben was outdoors. From what I found out, the hypnotist was definitely an amateur. When I talked with Dr. Trippe, we agreed to wait until we had an answer to our letter.

I had learned not to discourage Ben in anything he wanted to do that he thought might help him to regain speech, unless it was something that could hurt him. He had too many other frustrations.

"Shield the aphasic patient against frustration," I remembered having read in a pamphlet; and thought of a woman friend whose mother had aphasia and limited use of her right hand.

The mother had been a successful painter in oils before her stroke. She lived with her daughter. One day the daughter went to her mother's room and found her laying out paints. She was tempted to stop her. What would it do to the mother to learn that she could no longer paint? Or would it do more harm not to let her try?

When the mother looked up, her eyes bright, the daughter said, "Can I help?"

The mother smiled, shook her head, and went on arranging her paints.

Later, when the daughter returned, the mother was looking at the landscape she had just finished. It might have been done by a six-year-old child. The daughter saw that she was not discouraged. Tomorrow, she would do better.

I often thought about that mother and daughter. How many failures and disappointments must we have before we make progress? What would have been the frustration of the mother if the daughter had stopped her? What would have been Ben's frustration if we had not written the letter to the hypnotist?

But this was different. What if the hypnotist thought, in spite of the fact that he was an amateur, that he could help Ben?

One morning I saw Ben take a letter from the mailbox. As he started down our driveway, I knew from the way he walked that *the* letter had come. He gave it to me to open. To prevent my hand from trembling as I used the letter opener, I braced my elbow on the table.

It consisted of only one sentence — "I am sorry, but I cannot help Mr. McBride."

I tried not to show my relief . . . but what had it done to Ben? The same words that he had read and heard so often. I couldn't tell what he was thinking, but he didn't look as dejected as I had seen him after other disappointments. Was he learning to accept them ... or, now that it was over, was he admitting that he had had his doubts about the hypnotist? I never learned what he thought. Again — if only we could have talked about it.

I was learning, and I felt that he, too, was learning to take our losses with our progress. The progress we had made since the stroke was so much greater than our losses that we had a lot to be thankful for.

He picked up the letter, read it again, laid it down, looked at the clock, got his hat and started to the barn. It was time for him to turn the cattle into the pasture with the pond.

Through the window I watched him open the gate for the cattle. I thought: one more entry for the progress side of the ledger. I would always be thankful for Ben's interest in his cattle. How many times had they helped him to forget frustrations?

When I saw Ben go into the barn, I telephoned Dr. Trippe to report the answer to our letter. "I am not surprised," he said.

"Then you thought an amateur hypnotist would know his limits?" Apparently he did but his next question made me forget the hypnotist ... "How's Ben? When is he coming in for his checkup?"

"I know his checkup is past due," I admitted, "but I haven't been able to get him in for it."

The checkup included treatment for fluid in the tissues, which meant hospitalization. Ben always had cooperated when it was time for a checkup. Had he refused this time because, for some reason or other, he did not want to go back to the hospital?

Dr. Trippe said, "Tell Ben that I want him at Research by three this afternoon."

"We'll be there," I promised. How I would get Ben to agree to go, I didn't know.

As I started to the barn to tell him, I heard the telephone extension in the cabin ringing. A friend said, "If you are going to be home this afternoon, we'll drive out." My answer to a prayer!

"Do come," I said. "Our doctor has just told me he wants Ben at Research by three for a checkup. I need your help to get him there." She knew we didn't drive.

Ben was not at the barn. I could see that he was not with the cattle in the front pastures, so I started toward the back pasture. Again and again I blew my whistle. No answer.

If the wind was in the wrong direction, sometimes he did not hear the whistle even if he was near. There was no wind, so he must have gone to the creek at the far end of the pasture. If so, he was too far away to hear my whistle.

I started toward the creek, all the time blowing the whistle. I was almost there when I heard his, "oh-oh!" I found him sitting on a rock beside the road from the creek.

No need to ask if he had been to the creek. I knew he was resting before he came back to the barn, and sat down beside him. I would not tell him about Dr. Trippe's order until we reached the barn. He needed all his strength for the walk back.

We sat on the rock for so long a time, I thought our friend would come to take us to the hospital before we were ready. Ben look so tired that I waited for him to make the first move.

Finally, he stood up and we started out. We were about halfway when I saw that he needed to rest again. We sat on the grass under a tall, old oak tree.

By the time we reached the barn, he had to rest again. We sat on the bench beside the big, sliding door.

After about five minutes (I knew I couldn't wait longer), I said, "Dr. Trippe wants you at Research by three this afternoon. Your checkup is past due."

When he did not respond, I wondered if he suspected that I had phoned? Maybe not. He knew that Dr. Trippe often called to ask how he was.

When he still sat, staring at the ground, I said, "It has been three months since your last checkup."

He stood up, checked the barn doors and walked toward the house. I wasn't sure that he had consented to go until I saw him get his electric razor and begin to shave. Had the walk to the creek made him realize he could not postpone the checkup any longer?

He was in the hospital nine days. His heart condition had worsened to the point that he would be compelled to sell his fourteen head of commercial cattle. I was concerned how he would take the news.

We had been home three days before I had the courage to say, "Dr. Trippe wants you to sell the cattle before cold weather. He thinks you should sell now. If we wait, it may take us into the winter to get them all sold."

He looked at me but I couldn't tell what he was thinking. Finally he wrote ... "CATTLE SELL RE-SISKED BUY."

I didn't know what "RESISKED" meant. He saw that I didn't and reached for a circular advertising a dispersal sale of registered Polled Herefords. I had seen him looking at the circular but thought it was only because he was interested in Polled Herefords. He knew we could not go to the dispersal sale even if it was not in another state.

He wrote again, "RESISKED BUY."

"You want to sell the cattle we now have and buy 'registered'?"

He nodded and wrote, "2 — 3 HEREFORDS POLLING."

"Two or three Polled Herefords." I was so relieved that he had been thinking about selling his cattle, I didn't stop to think what Dr. Trippe might say about two or three Polled Herefords. "So you have decided to go in for quality instead of quantity. It will be much easier to care for two or three through the winter."

He agreed and wrote . . . "GOLD MINE GOLD STRIKE." I couldn't think what he meant until I remembered that another city farmer in our area had stopped in and told us that Gold Strike, a son of the renowned bull, Gold Mine, was owned by a breeder to the north of us.

When Ben pointed to the north and then to the telephone, I said, "You want me to call the man who owns Gold Strike?"

He nodded and wrote, "2 — 3 COWS . . . GOLD STRIKE."

I started to say, "Shouldn't we wait until we sell the cattle we now have?" but changed my mind. If he had his Polled Herefords, it would make it easier to part with the fourteen commercial white face that he had spent so many happy hours with.

I telephoned the breeder and told him that my husband was interested in buying two or three registered Polled Hereford cows bred to Gold Strike.

He sent for us that evening. When we returned home, Ben was the happy owner of three registered Polled Hereford cows bred to Gold Strike.

The next day we listed our fourteen commercial white face by name. Ben wrote the price he wanted for each beside the name, and the price of the herd. I telephoned our ad to the newspaper.

A man who lived a few miles from us came to see the cattle. Ben met him at the door and brought him in to meet me. I explained Ben's loss of speech and told the man why we were selling the cattle; Ben would show him the herd.

From the window I watched Ben and the man drive the cattle into the barnyard. When Ben started to the house I knew he needed me.

The man asked our price for the herd. Ben wrote the price he had totaled. "Let's talk about it," I said to Ben, and explained to the man, "We want to check our figures. Will you excuse us for a few minutes?"

I must make certain that Ben was still satisfied with the price he had figured. After the stroke when he was re-learning to figure, we had made some unhappy mistakes.

We rechecked the price of each cow and calf . . . and the grand total. "Still okay?" I asked.

He nodded.

I made a copy of the listing and prices and he took it out to our prospective buyer. He read the list and said, "I'll take the herd."

I could hardly believe it! The entire herd! To our first prospect! I had thought we would have to sell them — perhaps in twos and threes . . . or even one at a time.

Ben and I looked at each other. I knew he was as surprised and happy as I . . . and a little sad. "They are all gentle," I said to the buyer when Ben walked to Bessie and rubbed her neck. "All pets."

"I see they are," the man said. "Don't worry — they

will have a good home with us."

When he reached for his check book, Ben wrote, "CASHER CHECK."

This, I did not know how to handle. I knew that farmers who had always lived in the community resented anybody who questioned their honesty . . . especially city farmers like us. What could I say?

I looked at the man and smiled. "Ben always asks for a cashier's check," I explained.

I held my breath until the man said, "That's okay. It's after bank hours now. I'll get a cashier's check in the morning and bring it when I come for the cattle about noon."

Ben pointed to the cattle chute that he had just built. I knew he wanted the man to see it, and said, "Ben would like to show you his new chute. Do you have time to see it?"

Before he could answer, Ben was leading him to the chute.

The next day, when the truck drove away with Bessie and her calf and all the other cows and calves, Ben and I watched as long as it was within sight.

I wanted to say, "We'll miss them," but said instead, "It has been fun but I know it is time for us to sell them."

Ben agreed and patted the pocket where he carried his billfold. "And a good investment," he seemed to say. I really hadn't figured how good the investment had been financially. For therapy, it had been perfect.

Ben wrote, "3 COWS."

I said, "They will be here tomorrow. Then we will have Gold Strike's sons and daughters to look forward to." When Ben smiled, I added, "Grandsons and granddaughters of Gold Mine."

That afternoon, a friend came. He brought a woman relative of his whom we had not met. She had never seen anyone who had lost his speech from a stroke and did not understand how it could happen. She knew other people who had had a stroke but not one had lost his speech.

She kept looking at Ben, who sat listening and silent until she said something he agreed with. He nodded and said, "Oh!"

"There!" she exclaimed. Before I could explain that Ben still had voice but his speech was limited to "oh" and two words, "mom" and "home," she said, "You can talk," and moved her chair closer to him. "Now say, 'I will talk.'"

Ben shook his head.

"Of course you can. You talked before the stroke. You can talk now."

The man who brought her looked embarrassed but he didn't seem to know what to say.

When she kept on telling Ben he could talk if he would try, I said, "It is not that simple. We have learned since Ben's stroke that loss of speech is not uncommon. Sometimes it returns in a few days or weeks. In Ben's case, the injury was more severe. We have had the best therapy available, but so far, all he has is 'oh'." I didn't add . . . and "mom" and "home." She would want to know if he could say "mom" and "home," why couldn't he say other things?

I was afraid if she didn't stop, I would lose my control and say something I'd regret. And how much longer could Ben take it? I said, "Let's go outside."

I didn't know what we would do outside but anything was better than this.

Ben and the man started toward the door but she did

not move. "Why don't you try sign language," she said, "like they have for the deaf and —."

Before she could say "dumb," I interrupted. "That would not work in our case."

She still looked unconvinced. I was glad when she started for the door. It would have done no good to try to explain to her why sign language was not for Ben. She would not understand his spelling problem.

Ben was already at the pasture fence, calling his "oh-oh!" for Sugar.

When the woman saw Sugar, she exclaimed, "A Tennessee Walker! Does Ben ride her?"

The man said, "You should see him ride."

"Would you like to ride?" I asked, first the woman and then the man.

The man thanked me and said, "It's time for us to go."

After they left, I waited to see if Ben would show any reaction. If he felt any resentment, he gave no sign. He picked up the circular advertising the sale of the registered Polled Herefords and was soon lost in it.

I was still wondering how the woman could be so thoughtless, but as I watched Ben, I thought: If he can forget, so can I.

We had not realized the difference in caring for fourteen head of cattle and looking after three cows. Ben enjoyed his free time. He spent hours studying Polled Hereford literature. I studied with him so I would know what he meant when he tried to tell me something: as when he wrote, "LAMPLICHTER," telling me that Rollette (the cow that would have Gold Strike's son) was of the Lamplighter line. He was so sure that Rollette would have a bull calf, I could only hope that he would not be disappointed.

He wrote "BBM — GOLD STRIKE," and I knew that was to be the calf's name. "A good name for a champion," I said.

His "oh-oh!" was so happy, I wondered how long he had been dreaming about registered Polled Herefords. I was glad that he now had them.

As the time for the arrival of BBM Gold Strike drew near, Ben spent most of his days with Rollette. When he wrote "VET," I knew he was telling me . . . if Rollette had any trouble, he wanted me to telephone for the veterinarian.

Only once had we called for help when a cow was calving. It was ten o'clock at night when we telephoned the veterinarian. He lived a short distance from us and arrived fifteen minutes after our call. The calf was already there. We learned not to be in a hurry to spend $7.50 for a service call. But Rollette was different.

Finally, we thought it was only a matter of hours until BBM would be with us. Ben shut Rollette in the barn and watched her all day. After dinner I stayed with him. The barn was bright with electric lights. We had comfortable seats on a bale of hay with another bale to our backs . . . but by ten-thirty I was tired and sleepy.

I looked at Rollette munching hay from the trough. "She's all right," I told Ben. "We need our rest."

Before he answered, he walked over and examined Rollette . . . then wrote "12 CLOCK."

"If you insist, I'll set the alarm for midnight, but you need a good night's sleep."

When he didn't answer, I said, "We need sleep more than Rollette needs us."

He looked at me, then wrote, "5:00 A.M."

"All right," I agreed, "I'll set the alarm for five."

✎ 10

Surgery – Hope for Speech?

The alarm woke me the next morning at five o'clock. It was a moment before I realized that Ben was not beside me. I looked out of the window and saw the floodlights were on in the yard.

From the window I saw the lights were on in the barn. Then I saw Ben go into the barn. I was slipping my dress on when I heard his "oh-oh-OH!" and knew the calf was here.

"Coming!" I called, grabbing my coat and zipping my dress on the way.

The barnyard was still dark. Ben came to meet me. The way he pressed my arm, I knew before we reached the barn the BBM was all that Ben had hoped for.

"Bully head!" I said. "Strong, straight legs."

Ben beamed and spread his hands over the calf . . . from head to rump. "Fancy general confirmation," I agreed.

"CHAMTION," he wrote.

"A champion, indeed!"

When BBM's half sister (the calf of one of the other cows bred to Gold Strike) arrived, Ben was happy but

136

she could not compare with BBM.

The two calves increased our herd to five. At the time Ben let me know that he wanted registered Polled Herefords, I was glad he wanted QUALITY. I was still glad, but I had not known that QUALITY cattle meant more expensive feed.

Our commercial white face had been fed cobmeal, hay and ordinary cattle salt. Now our feed bills were staggering. Ben showed no concern about the cost of the feed he ordered or how much he fed. I could have reminded him that a special characteristic of Polled Herefords was their ability to convert feed into beef economically. I said nothing. He enjoyed watching them eat.

When he wrote, "MOLASSAS," I knew he must mean molasses, but what did molasses have to do with cattle feed? I was glad when I telephoned the order to the feed company; they knew. They understood his aphasia.

The rest of his order was "CORN CRACK" for corn chops, "MEAL ROB" for cobmeal, and "MIN SALT" for mineral salt. So I ordered the amounts of each that Ben specified, and on delivery, wrote the check.

When I saw the bag of a dark brown, sticky mixture that smelled like molasses, I knew why Ben wrote, "MOLSSAS."

Feeding time was the big event of our day. I was given a box seat on a bale of hay so I could watch him measure and serve the feed. Then we sat together and enjoyed the cattle at their feeding trough.

It was the same every evening. Promptly on the hour, we started to the barn for our "Show," as we called it. When we took our seats on the bale of hay and the cattle began to eat and I saw the pride and joy on Ben's face, I thought, "What show on Broadway would we want to see night after night and always be thrilled?" I wanted to tell him that I was glad his hobby was something that was fun for both of us, and safe, but kept still. I avoided anything that might make him feel aphasia caused him to be different.

I knew a woman whose husband was a stroke patient. His hobby was unsafe — a workshop in his basement. Whenever he went to his workshop, she found some excuse to go to the basement so she could be there if he needed her.

His stroke had left him with coordination damage, and while he seldom used his power saw, she lived in terror of it. One time, when he started to use it and she stopped him, he was so thwarted that it was hours before he recovered.

I looked at Ben's contented cows and then at him. As he stroked the white crest on the back of BBM's neck, I said to myself, "— and contented man."

All through the autumn and early winter, he spent the greater part of his days with his Polled Herefords and the mare, Sugar. He no longer galloped her across the pasture, but whenever he wanted to go to the creek he rode her, or sometimes he led her into the yard, where he sat in a lawn chair and watched her eat bluegrass.

In the evening, we read or practiced writing and spelling. Ben was particularly interested in current events and world news, so we read those articles first.

Once, he gave me a magazine and pointed to a certain paragraph that he wanted me to read aloud. Little did I know the article would keep us busy for weeks!

The article summarized that present estimates are at least 175,000 Americans die of this medical accident (stroke) every year. In addition, 1.8 million now living have been disabled by it.

The magazine had come that day, but I had not seen the article. Ben didn't make a sound and did not move until I read the last word. Then his "oh-oh!" rang out with such enthusiasm that I was sorry I did not know what he was trying to tell me.

I had marveled at the expression he could put into his "oh!" and at how much he could make others, as well as me understand; however, I had no idea what he was trying to tell me when he kept pointing to the article.

Playing for time, I said, "I did not realize that so many people had strokes. Maybe now more will be done to help us."

When he pointed to his mouth, I said, "I wonder, too, how many have aphasia."

I could see that something else was on his mind when he wrote, "LETTER."

"Letter? You want to write to the author of the article?"

Ben shook his head, pointed to me, to himself, and then to the article. I still did not understand — until he gave me a pencil and notebook, picked up his own note pad and pencil, and wrote, "BOOK."

"You want us to write a book about what you and I have learned about strokes and aphasia . . . something that will help other stroke patients and their families?"

His entire face smiled. I knew before he nodded that it was what he wanted. I almost said, "We better start with an article before we try a book," but instead quickly changed my thought into a question, "Shall we begin now?"

He nodded and motioned for me to sit beside him on the sofa so we could see each other's notes.

He waited for me to begin. Everything had happened

so unexpectedly that it was a moment before I could ask,
"Shall we start by writing everything we can remember
we have learned by trial and error? The 'Do's' and the
'Don'ts'? We can organize our notes later and make an
outline."

He nodded in agreement.

"What would you suggest for the patient who is in bed
or in a wheel chair?"

"BIRDS," he wrote, and added, "FROWERS" (flowers).

"Good! If the patient is in bed he can watch the birds
and flowers from his window. If he is confined to a
wheelchair, he can go outdoors."

Ben again nodded.

"We would enjoy studying birds when we have time," I
added. He smiled. I knew he was thinking about the
books on birds which we hadn't had time to read.

"STARS," he wrote.

"A telescope and a new world. Something else for you
and me when we have time."

"Time," I thought as we smiled at each other, "when
you can break away from BBM."

"Isn't it wonderful to have so many things that we want
to do?" I said. He pointed to our books and I added,
"We never have time to read all we want to."

When the days grew shorter and colder, I was thankful
we had the book to work on. Ben was seldom outdoors
except for feeding the cattle. As I did my housework, I
made notes for the book. I knew that Ben was thinking
about the book, too, when he was feeding the cattle. He
often came back with suggestions he had written in his
notebook.

The evening when he came from the barn, his eyes

bright, I knew something good had happened. He gave me his notebook and pointed to a word he had written, "EUREKA."

"Eureka?" I repeated.

He nodded and wrote, "GREEK FENCE WIRE."

I was still trying to figure out what he wanted to tell me when he brought the dictionary and turned to, "eureka" meaning, "I have found it!"

"EUREKA," Ben wrote again while I marveled that so often he was able to spell unusual words correctly but still jumble the letters in many simple words.

"Eureka," I repeated aloud, "I have found it!" I could see he was happy that I was on the right track. "Have you found something?"

He grabbed his pencil and wrote, "FENCE WIRE HAY."

"You mean you found the roll of wire fencing that has been lost for so long?"

He beamed and nodded, then again wrote "HAY."

"You found it back of the bales of hay? But where? Not in the barn?" It had been cleared when the bales of new hay were stored last fall.

"SHEP," he wrote and changed to "SHED."

"In the old shed?" I had forgotten there was any hay in the shed. The way he grinned I guessed that he, too, had forgotten.

When he wrote "EUREKA" again and pointed to his notes for our book, I knew he had not only a title for the book but also the theme.

He was watching me, trying to read my thoughts. "Wonderful!" I said. "You have named our book. How can we list all we have found since your stroke?"

"FRIEH," he wrote.

I did not know what he meant and was afraid to guess when he was so happy. "Friends?" I ventured.

He smiled and nodded.

"Indeed we have found friends, both new and old, whose loyalty amazes us."

We spent a half hour remembering friends who came to see us when our drive was so drifted with snow that they had to pull off the highway at our gate, leave their cars and walk down to our house. Friends who came in the summer heat and shared picnics on the cabin porch.

People who stopped in for a short visit, and others who came on business, some of whom we had not met before, often said when they left, "We did not mean to stay so long but we have enjoyed *talking* with you."

Ben was looking at me over his notebook, waiting for me to add to the list of things we had found.

"Can we say that we have developed a sense of humor?"

His smile told me what I already knew . . . we had a long way to go yet. We had been so confused after the stroke, we had lost our sense of humor. After we saw how much it helped to ease tensions, we tried to see the funny side whenever we could. Sometimes when my attempt to be funny fell flat, I knew from the expression on Ben's face that he gave me "E" for effort.

When he started again to write, I thought, we could add *selflessness*. In doing for each other, we had learned to forget self.

The he showed me what he had written. "GOD." When he looked at me I knew we were thinking together, "It would take a chapter to tell how God had helped us to meet challenge after challenge."

As our notes for the book increased, we spent more time writing. I didn't know how to begin the book but when I saw that he wanted to get on with the actual writing, I said, "What would you think of our making a list of things we've learned that will help the stroke patient, especially those with aphasia . . . and his family? We might make two lists . . . 'DO'S' and 'DON'TS'?"

Before I finished, he drew a line down the center of a sheet of paper.

" 'DO'S' first?"

He nodded.

"Okay."

"No. 1 . . . It is important that the aphasic patient has therapy as soon as possible after the stroke. During the early months he will benefit more than at any other time.

"No. 2 . . . If he is an adult, treat him as an adult. He resents being treated as a child. (Ben nodded emphatically on this point.) The aphasic patient's problem is to learn how to communicate what he knew before the stroke, and lost.

"No. 3 . . . Help the patient to find a hobby, anything that will interest him. (When I made this suggestion, Ben wrote 'CATTLE' . . . and I said, 'Cattle is your hobby, but each patient must choose his own.')

"No. 4 . . . If the patient has lost his speech, ask questions that can be answered by nodding or shaking his head. Or, if he has limited speech, by 'yes' or 'no'.

"No. 5 . . . Allow him to do whatever he can for himself and encourage him.

"No. 6 . . . If the patient shows fatigue, suggest a rest period.

"No. 7 . . . It helps the aphasic patient and his family to meet other aphasics and their families. He sees he is not alone. Other people have problems too, some like his, some different. No two patients are alike nor do they make the same progress.

"No. 8 . . . Keep the patient one of the family, consult with him and ask his opinion. If he has neither his speech nor writing, you can ask, 'Would you do it this way' or 'that way?' until he shakes his head, or nods.

"No. 9 . . . It is most important that the patient relearns to write and spell. It takes time and patience, but is well worth every moment spent on it. Even without speech, if he has writing and spelling, he can communicate."

I stopped to see if Ben was tired. He wasn't, so I said, "Now the 'DON'TS'?"

He nodded.

"No. 1 . . . Don't hurry the patient." (Ben smiled and nodded, I wondered if he was remembering the time a friend phoned and asked us to go to church with him. He would stop by for us in twenty minutes. We were ready, but Ben was so exhausted from hurrying, I didn't know whether we should go or not. We went, but I learned — never again to accept an invitation unless we had plenty time to get ready for it).

"No. 2 . . . Avoid frustrating the patient. Do not scold or argue with him."

Ben nodded and smiled.

"No. 3 . . . Don't interrupt the patient when he is trying to say or write something."

Again Ben nodded and smiled. I said, "This next suggestion will help the patient when he starts to regain speech."

"No. 4 . . . If the patient repeats words and phrases over and over, or if he says 'No' when he means, 'Yes', or 'Yes' when he means 'No', be careful how you correct him. You may only confuse him.

"No. 5 . . . Don't force the patient to meet people or into strange situations until he is ready." Ben smiled and I said, "That doesn't mean you. You are always ready to meet anybody — or anything."

He nodded and looked at the clock. "It's time to feed BBM and Rollette," I agreed.

He patted our notebooks and I knew he was saying, "Good work. A good start on our book." But there was something he wanted to add before he went to the barn. "PALN," he wrote.

"Plan?" I asked. "You want to tell the patient it helps to plan each day?" He nodded, and I said, "We not only plan each day but we set definite goals. Shall we say, 'A definite goal within his ability gives the patient a purpose to his life?'" He agreed and I said, "We'll list it under the 'DO'S'."

After dinner, I thought he might want to resume our work on the book, but was glad when he picked up a magazine that had come that day. We needed a rest period.

Before I finished the dishes, he showed me an article that made us forget everything else. Here was another hope for speech.

Ben had underscored the lines that told how Dr. Michael E. DeBakey of the Texas Medical Center in Houston, Texas, which is associated with Baylor University's College of Medicine, had found that stroke may stem from a clotting process in arteries leading to but actually outside of the brain . . . in the carotid artery, a blood vessel running through the neck — within reach of the blood vessel surgeon.

Ben's face was bright with hope as he pointed to the telephone.

"You want me to call Dr. Trippe and ask him what he thinks about it for you?"

He nodded so emphatically, I knew he wanted the surgery. Could his heart stand surgery? If it could and speech returned — but the article said that surgery was more successful soon after the stroke and it had been almost six years since Ben's stroke. What would another failure do to him?

Then there was the chance that the clot was not in the neck artery but in the brain. And if in the artery, which artery?

"Ben," I said, "you understand that the surgeon will first inject dye into the artery and take an X-ray picture. If a clot shows, he will remove it and —."

He nodded and again pointed to the telephone. As I dialed, I knew that if Dr. Trippe said it was safe and recommended a neurosurgeon, Ben would be in the hospital as soon as a room was available.

He was hospitalized the next day.

11

A New Low

The waiting room of the hospital was quiet. Our prayers were with our loved ones in surgery. Whenever steps sounded in the hall, all eyes turned to the door. One by one the family physician or surgeon came with his report.

Finally, Ben's neurosurgeon stood before me. "Your husband has a perfect artery," he said. He was telling me that the X-ray showed no clot in the dye treated artery. What a kind way to break the news, I thought. Another hope for speech had failed.

How can I tell Ben? I wondered. He was so hopeful that his loss of speech was not from brain injury but from a clot in the artery, and that the clot could be removed, and that he would talk again.

I said, "Is he all right?"

"Yes. I promised you I would take no chances. When he started to show a reaction, we did not do the other artery."

"He doesn't know?"

"Not yet. We gave him a general. He won't know anything for an hour or two."

147

"Then I will go back to his room and wait for him," I said. "Thank you for trying — and not taking any chances."

When they brought Ben back to his room his eyes were closed. I was glad. If he could sleep I would have more time to think how to tell him.

I saw his eyelids quiver and thought, "He is afraid to open his eyes. The longer he doesn't ask, the longer he can hope." Then he opened his eyes, wide and questioning.

"You are all right, dear," I said, and heard myself quoting the neurosurgeon, "You have a perfect artery." For a moment I hoped that he might still be hazy from the anesthetic and would not realize what the words meant.

As he closed his eyes again, I knew from the expression on his face that he understood. Afraid to trust my voice, I laid my hand on his. For an hour I watched him. The nurse checked regularly. "It's the anesthetic," she said. I knew better.

When he did open his eyes, he looked out of the window at the setting sun. I knew he was telling me that I should start home. He worried if I was not there before dark. I had always telephoned him as soon as I had arrived.

"I'm glad you are awake," I said. "I knew you would want me to leave so I could be home before dark but I couldn't go while you were asleep."

He looked at the telephone on his bedside table. He was telling me to call a cab *now*.

"I'm going in just a minute," I told him as I pulled a chair close to his bed and took his hand in mine. One — two — three, I tapped gently. I could barely feel his one

— two — three as he answered with his thumb but his eyes said, "I love you."

"I love you too," I whispered, and kissed his forehead.

His eyes followed me to the door.

He was in the hospital a week. Dr. Trippe kept him there for a rest and to check his heart.

It was near the end of the week the day I learned he was to have a new night nurse (he always had had the same around-the-clock nurses). I was glad she came on duty in time for me to meet her before I left the hospital. I wanted to explain Ben's writing — how he sometimes misspelled words or how he might write only the first letters of a word.

Before I had a chance to tell her anything about his writing, Ben looked out of the window and pointed to the telephone. "I know it's getting late," I said. "I'm going just as soon as I tell your nurse about your Polled Herefords." There wasn't time to explain Ben's writing, but if she knew about his prized bull calf, he could show her his snapshots of the calf and its mother.

"I'm a farmer, too," the nurse said. "My husband and I raise cattle in Platte County."

Ben's eyes brightened. "Platte County!" I said. "That's where we live. What kind of cattle do you raise?"

"Angus."

Ben smiled as he shook his head and reached into the drawer of his bedside table for the pictures of his Polled Herefords. "You two will get along," I said, as Ben handed her the picture of BBM. "That's his champion bull calf, grandson of the world famous Gold Mine."

They'll get along all right, I reassured myself as I rode the elevator down to the lobby to wait for my cab. I stopped worrying.

The next morning I found Ben flushed and dazed. I took one look and went to find his nurse.

Before I could ask what was wrong, she said, "Ben had a little trouble last night. He is still under sedation."

"Trouble? What kind of trouble? He was all right when I left yesterday."

"He had indigestion . . ."

"And wanted an Alka-Seltzer," I said. "You would have known what his 'ALKA' meant. The new nurse didn't get it?"

"No. She brought him an apple, and he blew his top."

"Was anyone hurt?"

"No," the nurse said and smiled. "I don't know what happened to the apple. He threw it and broke a vase of flowers on the dresser."

"But nothing like this ever happened before."

"We understand him," the nurse said.

I went back to Ben's room and stood in the doorway, watching him. He gave no sign he knew I was there. I saw Dr. Trippe at the desk in the hall, and walked over to him.

"Ben had a little indigestion last night," he said.

"Yes, I know."

"He is finding it hard to accept his disappointment in the dye test."

"If he could only talk about it," I said.

Dr. Trippe didn't answer and I saw that he had something else on his mind. Finally he said, "I think Ben should sell his cattle."

"He sold the fourteen commercial white face, you know. All he has now are his five registered Polled Herefords. If he has to sell his prized bull calf —." I stopped. "Of course, you know best."

"Ben needs more rest," he said. "He might keep the calf and mother for awhile. We'll see how he gets along."

"I'll help with the feeding," I promised.

"Ben worries if he thinks you are working too hard."

"I know. I'll be careful. How soon do you want him to sell the other three?"

"We'll give him two weeks to rest after he goes home."

Ben had been home from the hospital two weeks but still seemed tired and apathetic. He sat for hours looking out of the windows. Was it because he had been so sure there was a clot that could be removed and he would regain speech?

He was weaker and I worried that it might be from the dye test, but was assured that it was not. I knew his heart ailment had worsened. That was why Dr. Trippe wanted him to sell the two cows and heifer. I had not told Ben about selling the cattle. First, I must bring him out of his dejection. Would a suggestion that we continue work on our book help?

I doubted now that we would be able to write a book, but I would not tell him so. We would keep on making notes. At the right time, I might ask if he would like to try an article first. It would be quicker and we could still work on the book.

One morning after he picked up a magazine, turned the pages and laid it down, I said, "We already have enough notes to write an article. Would you like to do a 1500 to 2000 word piece while we are gathering material for the book?"

I saw a flicker of interest.

"The article might help us sell the book."

He smiled but didn't say anything. He was interested in writing but had found time to write only one article. It

sold to *Nation's Business.* What would be his reaction if
"Eureka" did not sell? I wouldn't worry. The important
thing now was for him to have a new interest to replace
the cattle he must sell.

We spent the rest of the day selecting material from our
notes and making an outline for the article.

That evening while he was feeding the cattle, I telephoned Dr. Trippe. "I know you said we'd give Ben two
weeks after he came home from the hospital before
telling him to sell part of his cattle, but he has been
feeling so low, I couldn't say anything until I found
another interest for him. I've found it."

"Good! What is it?"

"We're writing an article."

"What about?"

"Aphasia."

"We'll wait one more week, but no longer. I don't want
Ben feeding too many cows this winter."

We worked on the article every morning. I was happy
to see Ben's interest grow. Finally I had to say, "Dr.
Trippe wants you to sell all the cattle except BBM and
Rollette."

He gave no sign he heard me. I was trying to think
what to say next when he snapped his thumb and
forefinger, asking — now?

"Yes. I am glad you can keep BBM and Rollette." He
nodded. From the expression on his face, I thought —
He is not surprised. He knows he is growing weaker.

We advertised them the next day. He wrote the price he
wanted for each cow and the heifer — and the total for the
three.

Our first prospects were professional lookers. We
expected them. We knew it was not easy to sell registered

cattle from a small herd. Breeders of registered cattle usually could afford large herds and had their own markets.

It was late afternoon before our real prospects came. When they started to look at BBM and Rollette, I explained they were not for sale. Then Ben showed the men the two cows and heifer he advertised.

Ben pointed to the head of each, and I knew what he wanted me to say. "Polled Herefords, as you know, are naturally hornless. They are born that way and horns never develop."

Ben pointed to the hind quarters of each animal and I said, "Polled Herefords grow more beef." I felt foolish telling these men things they already knew — better than I — but when I paused I could see that Ben wanted me to say more. I tried to remember what I had read and quoted — "Polled Herefords have the ability to convert feed into beef more economically and more efficiently than most beef cattle."

Ben nodded and I knew I was doing all right so far. Again he pointed to the head of each cow and the heifer, and again I quoted: "The head of a Polled Hereford has good, prominent polls."

I was glad when the men walked over to the heifer and began their own appraisal.

Finally Mr. Adams, the spokesman, said, "We will give you for the three — " and named a figure slightly under Ben's price.

Ben shook his head.

"We will send our truck for them," Mr. Adams said.

Ben wrote "VET" and pointed to himself. He was saying he would have the expense of.the veterinarian's health check on each animal before it left the farm.

The men held a conference; then Mr. Adams turned to Ben and smiled, "You win."

As he counted out in cash Ben's price, I said to myself, "Thank goodness, I don't have to ask for a cashier's check."

With only BBM and Rolette to look after, we had more time to work on our article, but we accomplished little. I didn't know whether he had lost interest, whether he missed the cattle, or whether it was because he was too tired. The article was not finished. Later I rewrote it and sold it under the title, "Silence Was Golden" to *Together* magazine.

Our days were quiet. Ben did only necessary chores, and I kept my time free to read to him or do anything I thought might interest him.

When he came in after feeding BBM and Rollette one morning, I could see that he was having trouble breathing, and telephoned Dr. Trippe. He ordered a small, hand-operated oxygen tank. It gave some relief, but he still had difficulty. Evenings were the worst. When he wrote, "SURELY" one night, it was a few minutes before I knew what he was trying to say. "Yes, it is sultry," I agreed. "You will feel better when the weather changes."

He shook his head.

I tried to think of something to cheer him. A few days before, the mail had brought pictures in color that we had taken of BBM. Ben was happy with the calf's development.

I brought out the pictures now and gave them to Ben. "His color is perfect," I said.

While he was looking at the pictures of BBM, I took another picture from the envelope . . . of Ben and a friend taken late in the summer. I was startled at the change I saw in Ben — and that was last summer. He looked almost as thin and haggard as he did now. Why hadn't I realized it when the pictures came? Had Ben seen it?

He gave me the pictures of BBM, lay back and closed his eyes. I watched him until I thought he was asleep, then went to my desk. I had letters that must be written.

I didn't know he was awake until I heard him say, "Oh!"

When I saw that he was writing, I was glad that some interest had awakened him. He gave me the notepad and I read, "SUCDICE." I knew what he meant but refused to admit it.

He took the pad back and wrote, "SUCICDE."

I studied the letters but still would not admit that I understood what he was trying to say.

He tried again, "SUIDICE."

As our eyes met, I saw that he realized I knew what he had written in his own way . . . SUICIDE.

ᵓ 12

Legal Advice

I looked at the word Ben had tried to write . . . "SUICIDE," and wanted to say, "Ben, you don't mean that." But he did mean it. Now that he knew his heart was failing, life without hope was not worth fighting for. He who had devoted so many years to helping others thought he was through.

I took his hand in mine and said, "Ben, I need you."

He smiled, and as his hand tightened over mine, I knew he would give me the last ounce of his strength.

"We don't know why you lost your speech, but we do know we have grown closer to God and closer to each other these past six years. Because we have been living one day at a time and trusting Him, He has not let anything happen to us that He has not seen us through."

Silence. What more could I say?

Finally, Ben wrote, "JOB."

Often he had written "Job," or had given me the Bible, opened to the Book of Job.

I said, "Yes, I know. Job wished for death when his afflictions were more than he could bear, but — ." Ben brought the Bible. I was to read how God helped Job.

I prayed that I would turn to the verse Ben needed. We had underscored so many verses in past reading, which should I choose?

Chapter 23, verse 10, was underscored and double checked. I read, "But he knoweth the way that I take: when he hath tried me, I shall come forth as gold."

Ben motioned for me to read on . . . "My foot hath held his steps, his way have I kept, and not declined."

There was no need to read more. From the expression on Ben's face, I knew the tension had eased.

The next day I could feel a new serenity in him. When he looked at me across the breakfast table, I thought, "He wants me to know . . . last night he was at the end of his rope, but he is all right now."

What could I say to let him know I understood? I decided not to say anything. We would have a happy day, as if nothing had happened last night.

The sun was trying to break through the clouds. I suggested that, perhaps later in the day, it would be warm enough for us to take a short walk before feeding time.

There was no warming. After a half-hearted effort, the sun gave up and the clouds took over. Ben stepped outside long enough to satisfy himself that we would have to make our own warmth inside. He came back with logs for the fireplace.

When he set up the card table before the fire, I waited to see what he would do. He brought out a plat of Lawn Acres and pointed to the lot we had reserved for ourselves. For a moment I thought, "Is he thinking we should sell or lease the farm now, and build in Lawn Acres?"

That couldn't be it. He had let me know that he would

never leave the farm. Even if I should die first, he meant to stay on. He would finish the cabin and rent it to a retired couple . . . hire the man to help him with the cattle and chores . . . and the man's wife could clean his house once a week and prepare his dinners. He could manage breakfast and lunch.

When he again pointed to our lot on the plat and looked at me, I thought he was trying to say . . . If he should go first, I was to sell or lease the farm and build a house in Lawn Acres. We had talked about that, too.

Until now it had been easy to talk about our plans in case one of us should be left alone. Today, the little house in Lawn Acres seemed too close to realization to talk about.

I was thinking how to change the subject when he wrote, "CITSERN."

"You ended our water problem when you had the cistern dug," I said.

He smiled, and I wondered if he was remembering how long it had taken me to understand what he meant the first time he tried to write "cistern." First it was "CIRTIN" — then "CITSERN." Not until he wrote, "RAINY WATER," and drew a picture of a tank, did I know.

We had needed a cistern. The well with its rock wall that had served us all the years we had lived at the farm now leaked. We were having water hauled regularly to add to the well supply which furnished running water to our house. Expensive, but within our budget.

A new cistern would mean a big cash outlay, and I knew nothing about its construction. Where would we find a contractor? And how could Ben make him understand what he wanted?

Ben had no fear. As a teen-ager he had helped his father

dig and finish a cistern. He could do it again. He wrote, "4000 GAL" for capacity; "COMCRET" for concrete; and "COLECATE" for charcoal filter.

We found a contractor who understood what Ben wanted. Together, they decided where to dig the cistern — near the northeast corner of the house. In record time a 4000-gallon cistern with guttering and a charcoal filter, and a new jet pump in the basement, were completed. Ben was happy. So was I.

I said, "You amaze me the way you work with total strangers and make them understand what you want. Do you know how many have told me that you work harder than they do?"

He shook his head, and I thought from the expression on his face that he was thinking, "I can't do it now."

"I remember something else you did that surprised me." He wanted to know what it was.

"The time you wired the barn for lights."

He smiled and waited to hear more.

"That day when the Power and Light Company set the new pole in the south pasture and you let the workmen know that if they were going to discard the old pole, you would like to have it."

His smile widened.

"When they said you could have it, you led one of the workmen to the barn lot and showed him where you wanted to use the pole."

Ben nodded, his eyes bright — remembering.

"Two of the men carried the pole to the barn lot and left it on the spot you pointed out. I knew then that your next project would be to wire the barn for lights."

He smiled and motioned with his hands as if measuring wire.

"You managed that, too. The workmen gave you the old wire along with the pole. The next thing I knew, you and Jess (his part-time helper at the farm) had the pole set and were wiring the barn."

He looked so happy, I said, "When did you learn electric wiring?"

He grinned and tapped his head. I remembered his having told me that he helped his father wire the house when they dug the cistern.

"Jess got a kick out of your telling him how to do wiring," I said. "You even planned it so we can turn on the lights at the barn from the house."

He wasn't listening, but looking out of the window toward the barn. I thought, "Is he remembering the night when all the lights at the barn were on as we awaited the arrival of BBM?"

A shadow crossed his face and I wondered if he was worrying about what would happen when he couldn't do the outside chores. What could I say to cheer him?

I smiled and said, "I certainly made it rough for you when you tried to do something and you couldn't make me understand what it was. Remember the time you wanted to cut the brush out of the fence rows and tried to tell me you needed a machete?"

He smiled with me.

"You worked so hard writing 'machete', it's a wonder you didn't give up cutting the brush. It took you more than an hour to make me understand what a machete is."

He nodded and I said, "Just for fun, let's look in your notebook and see how many ways you wrote it before I finally got it. I know where to find it."

He looked doubtful.

"It's in notebook No. 3 — I think it's the page with

the corner turned down."

After I found it, I wished I hadn't. Would it discourage him to see how far off his spelling had been — and would he realize there had not been as much improvement in his spelling as we had hoped for?

At first, we had worked hard on correcting his spelling — only to learn that too often he forgot, and the next time he wrote the word, it still was misspelled.

I was glad now when I saw his amusement as we read about machete . . . his "MESSCLICATTE . . . MESSIL-TACETEC . . ." and finally . . . "CUBA . . . MICEL-TATE . . . ARMY NAVY STORE."

He didn't seem discouraged, so I said, "And still I didn't get it — not until you brought the dictionary. There it was — 'machete' — with two illustrations; one machete short and broad, the other long and not so wide, with the definition, 'A large, heavy knife used esp. in South America and the West Indies, for cutting cane, clearing paths, etc.' and 'for use as a weapon'."

Ben took the notebook and began to look through it. He didn't know that I had kept a list of his misspelled words: 992 of them.

So that he wouldn't be too disheartened, I said, "We should have a record of the thousands of words you spell correctly. They far outnumber your misspellings." He deserved credit for his writing and spelling effort.

When he started his writing exercise by making a series of circles for arm movement, I said, "Everyone who has lost his speech from a stroke should learn to write and spell." He nodded emphatically. "We can't count all the happy hours we've had from your writing."

He nodded and turned to a page in the notebook we would long remember. "RECKINMITSIC . . . RICH-

RAMROS ... PIANO." Then ... "SOPLORMO ...
HIHT SCHOOL ... OFERO ... URICHT."

I laughed. "That day, without speech, you told me
something I had not known about you after all the years
we had been together."

He nodded and smiled.

"When you were a sophomore in high school, you
worked as an usher at the Convention Hall. You heard
the best known operas and musicians, including Rachmaninoff."

He was living it over again.

"Remember how we got out the encyclopedia and the
wonderful time we had, reading about famous musicians?" And so the day passed. Though it was cold and
cloudy outside, inside we were happy before the warm
fireside — remembering.

The next day the sun was bright, but the wind was
chilling. We were out only long enough to do the chores
at the barn. As so often happened, a happy day was
followed by one that was not. This was an unhappy day.

At breakfast, I saw that Ben had a faraway look in his
eyes. Perhaps he had had a bad dream and would forget
it. Whatever it was that troubled him was still there when
he left the breakfast table and went to the living room.

He waited until I finished washing the dishes, then
motioned for me to sit beside him on the sofa.

"DIE," he wrote ... "AURLOSY ... DR."

I knew what he meant. If the doctors could learn
anything from his brain that would help others regain
speech, he wanted an autopsy. How should I answer?

Finally I said, "Are you telling me — you want Dr.
Trippe to ask for an autopsy after —?" I was glad he
nodded before I had to say more.

When he pointed to his mouth, and then to his head, I said, "They may be able to learn something that will help others who have lost their speech; that's what you want?"

He nodded again. So that was what he had been thinking about. Now, maybe, he would stop worrying. But there was something else. What?

I knew when he pointed to his eyes. It was a moment before I could say, "You want to leave your eyes to the Lion's Eye Tissue Bank of the University of Missouri?"

He nodded. When I could trust my voice, I said, "I want to leave my eyes, too. We'll check to see what we must sign."

He seemed satisfied, but it was time we talked about something else. I thought about our article, "Eureka." We had agreed not to send it out again until after the first of the year, but we might read it and see if we could do anything to improve it.

Suddenly he looked very tired, and I knew it was time for him to rest. I said, "I don't know why I'm so sleepy. Shall we take a nap?"

He stretched out on the sofa and closed his eyes. I went to our bedroom.

When I returned to the living room, he was reading Francis Bacon *(Essays* and *New Atlantis)*. He pointed to the lines he had underscored — "It is true greatness to have in one the frailty of a man, and the security of a God."

This time it was I who nodded. I couldn't trust myself to speak.

The next day started off happy. It was warmer. Ben stepped outside to test the weather. When he came back he nodded and pointed to the barn. He was telling me . . . it was warm enough, we could stay out for awhile after we fed BBM and Rollette. He was remembering Dr. Trippe's order — not to stay out too long when the weather was cold or windy.

It was a wonderful half hour. We returned to the house, happy and warmed by the sunshine. I had gone to the mailbox and had a handful of Christmas cards from friends — all with personal messages. Many said, "Hi, Ben! Good to see you writing again."

When we finished reading the cards, Ben wanted to work on the cards we were sending. I had addressed them and had written a note on each, ready for Ben's and my signatures. He enjoyed signing them but writing soon tired him, so we did only a few at a time.

In the mail that day was a card from a friend who was recovering from a stroke. He was one of those fortunate people who lost speech but regained it in a few days. He still had trouble with his writing.

Ben was so touched by Frank's card, he wanted to answer it. I wrote a short personal note which Ben copied and signed. He made several mistakes in the copying but I said nothing. Frank would understand.

The weather continued mild for mid-December. Ben and I chose the late afternoon for feeding time. BBM and Rollette were always waiting for us.

That day when Ben took Rollette's head between his hands, I knew he was trying to tell her something. Before we left the barn lot, he went to Rollette and stroked her neck; then he turned to BBM. He looked at the calf a long time. I tried to think of something to say. Before I could say anything, he turned and walked toward the house. When I caught up with him, I saw that he was having difficulty with his breathing.

As soon as we were in the house, he lay down on the

sofa and closed his eyes. I watched him as I addressed more Christmas cards.

An hour later, he sat us and reached for his notepad. I waited until he finished writing and brought the notepad to me.

"SICK," I read . . . "WILLIS" (wills) . . . "LAWER" (lawyer) . . . "BANK."

I knew what he meant. We had talked of adding a codicil to our wills (written in 1954) so as to make our bank the executor, but had never got it done. Was he strong enough to take a cab to the city to our lawyer's office, or should I ask the lawyer to come to us?

While I was trying to think what to say, he again wrote "BANK." Of course! We would have to go to the bank. Our wills were in the lock box there. Our lawyer would need all three copies.

Ben pointed to the telephone, and I said, "If we can get an appointment for tomorrow, shall we go in?"

He nodded.

"Perhaps we should," I agreed. "This good weather can't last."

The next morning we could feel the change in the weather but we called a cab and went to the city.

It started to snow while we were at the lawyer's office. As soon as we signed the codicil, Ben looked out of the window at the fast-falling snow.

"I'll call a cab from the bank as soon as we leave our copies of the wills in the lock box," I promised.

Our home was only twelve miles north of the city but we found with every mile, the snow was deeper. When the cab turned off the highway into our drive, the snow was beginning to drift. We were glad we had not waited longer to start home.

As the driver let us out at our house, he said, "Merry Christmas. Looks like it's going to be white."

"Merry Christmas," I returned, "to you and yours." Ben clasped his hand.

We watched the cab plow its way through the drifted drive back to the highway. When Ben turned to me, I knew he was thinking with me: If this keeps up we soon will be snowbound.

13

Snowbound

As I stepped into the house, I sighed with relief. So good to be home! I could feel its warmth reach out and enfold me. Did Ben feel it, too? But where was Ben?

Then I saw him at the closet where he kept his sheepskin coat, cap and boots. He was pulling on his boots. Yes, he was glad to be home — in time to do the feeding before dark.

I started to say, "Wait a minute and I'll go with you," then remembered that the barn was his special province. How much longer would he be able to feed his cattle? If the snow kept up, I knew what Dr. Trippe would say. "Ben, you are NOT to go out in this snow."

I said, "I'll have the soup ready when you come back and a fire burning in the fireplace." The day before we had made beef-vegetable soup and stored it in the refrigerator for tonight. I had laid only three small logs for the fireplace. We would be too tired after our day in the city to stay up late.

As Ben walked to the barn I watched from a window. There was no path. Not even the driveway to the barnyard showed. From the house to the barn, it was as

167

though a huge, white sheet had been stretched tight with only shrubs and trees showing through. When he reached the 10-foot gate into the barnyard, I wondered if the snow was already so deep that he would have trouble pushing the gate open. He shoved it aside just enough to wedge through.

The next morning when I woke, I saw Ben standing at a window, looking out. He motioned for me to join him and reached for my hand.

Overnight our little world had been transformed. The trees were snow-capped, and each branch wore its own artistry; the telephone and electric wires had been turned into pure white strands jeweled with crystal pendants; the fence between the yard and pastures was no longer ordinary mesh wire with some of the wires bent out of shape — instead, every wire was like tinsel — perfect in its mantle of snow. And the cabin! What magic held that massive overhang of snow from sliding off the roof of the porch?

"I have NEVER seen anything like it!" was all I could say.

Ben nodded and brought his camera. When he pointed to the thermometer outside the window, I knew he was telling me that it was warm enough to go outdoors and take pictures.

I agreed. "If we stay out of the deep snow."

The wind that had swept certain areas clean and piled the snow in drifts had died during the night, leaving the path to the cabin clear.

As we finished taking the pictures, the sky began to darken. Ben gave me the camera and went to the barn. If we were to have more snow, he wanted the feeding done.

I saw the mail carrier stop at our box on the highway.

When Ben came from the barn, I had a stack of Christmas cards waiting to be opened.

He recognized the return address on one of the cards and opened it first. It was from a friend we had not heard from in the past year.

Ben read the card, then reread it. When he gave it to me I knew something had happened to Les. A heart attack, I read. "Not Les."

Before Ben's strokes he had had a heart attack. After six months (three months in the hospital and at home, and another three months of limited time at the office) his recovery was satisfactory.

"Not Les," I said again.

But it was Les. "A heart attack four months ago." He had written, "I thought it would never happen to me. I guess I'm lucky to be alive but when they tell me I've still got to take it easy . . . Ben, I've thought of you so often. The progress you've made. Your courage. The way you've kept going . . ."

Ben gave me his tablet. While I was reading Les's card, he had written, "LETTER."

"We'll write Les as soon as we get in more wood." It had started to snow again. The logs for the fireplace were piled and covered with canvas in a protected corner of the porch. We laid logs on the grate and filled the fireside basket.

While we were bringing in the wood I knew Ben must be remembering his own heart attack and four strokes. He had followed doctor's orders when he had the heart attack. But the four strokes — four warnings. All unheeded.

In 1953, he had his first stroke. Because it was a little stroke, we ignored the warning. That morning he was lifting two 100-pound sacks of grain, one at a time, but when he dropped one sack and had to lift it again, that made three hundred pounds.

When he walked into the house a few minutes later, his face was drawn and his right arm hung at his side, useless.

He didn't go to the office that day but rested on the sofa. The next morning he could use his arm but he still looked tired. I thought he would stay home at least one more day, but when he came to breakfast, he was dressed for the office.

He saw my surprise, and before I could say anything, he explained — an out-of-town client was coming to the office that day to interview sales trainee applicants. I knew there was no use in my saying, "Let me take care of it for you." I had been working at the office for the past five years. Nor would he think his secretary could handle it for him.

His second stroke was in 1954. We had had an unusually busy day at the office. It was after five o'clock. Ben and I were alone. Before we went home he had to prepare for a meeting of the Kansas City Employment Board the next morning, and had asked me to get certain papers for him from the files.

When I took the papers to him he was slumped over his desk, unconscious. I telephoned Dr. Trippe. In minutes, an ambulance came to take him to the hospital. He had a private nurse that first night. And after that was in round-the-clock nursing a month. When he was released there was no apparent damage except his loss of vision to the left in both eyes.

That was our second warning, also ignored. Nor did we try to learn if medical science could tell us what to do to prevent another stroke.

The third stroke was so slight, we hardly noticed it. That was in 1955.

Then, on January 7, 1956, came the stroke that left him with aphasia. In a few more days it would be six years since he lost his speech.

He looked so depressed as we started our letter to Les, that I thought . . . he is remembering and wants to write something to Les to keep him from making the same mistakes we made.

I said, "Les will be able to learn more about heart attacks and strokes than we could in 1956."

Ben nodded.

"Medical science is discovering ways to detect early warnings and prevent strokes." I wondered if Ben was thinking . . . if only people will heed the warning. "Shall we send Les our clippings about strokes?" Before I could finish the question, Ben was on his way to our file where we kept the clippings.

After he gave them to me, he wrote, "DR. 6 MOS."

"Yes," I agreed, "Les should have regular checkups every six months. More often at first. He should take it easy until his doctor tells him he can go back to his office."

Ben smiled, and I knew, or perhaps I imagined, he was thinking: That's more than I did.

We had been so absorbed in our letter to Les, that, not until it was finished, did we realize how much snow had fallen in the last two hours. And it was still snowing. From our front window we watched it blowing and drifting in our driveway.

Ben walked to a window in the kitchen and looked toward the barn. We were glad the feeding had been done for the day, but what about tomorrow?

The next morning it had stopped snowing but when I looked at the gate to the barnyard, I knew Ben could not open it alone. Together we pushed and were able to get through.

The snow from the house to the gate was deep but in the barnyard it was even deeper . . . over our high boots.

I was afraid for Ben. When he stopped to rest, I said, "Won't you let me go on? My boots are higher than yours."

He didn't answer but started out again. When we reached the barn he sat down on a bale of hay. I sat beside him. It was warm in the barn. Bales of hay were stacked to the rafters on the north wall. On the floor beside us were several bales with their binding cords cut so it would be easy to transfer the hay to the mangers. I knew then why Ben had been so long at the barn the day before. In case there came a time when he could not do the feeding, there would be no bales of hay for me to lift and open.

He spread hay in the manger for BBM and Rollette. Then as he measured the grain for each animal, I watched so I would know just how much to give each.

I looked out of the barn window at our tracks from the gate and thought, "Going back will be easier."

But Ben was not ready to go back to the house. He had his ax and wanted to test the ice on the pond. If it was frozen deep enough to be safe for the cattle, he would cut a water hole. The gate to the pond was closed because last year a neighbor had lost six one-thousand-pound-steers when they broke through the snow-covered ice on his pond.

The snow didn't look deep down the slope to the pond

but Ben had had enough for one day. Especially if he decided to cut a water hole. What would be his reaction if I tried to stop him? How would I feel if he tried to stop me on something I wanted to do? But I had no heart problem. If he did start to chop the ice and collapsed at the pond — ?

Finally, I said, "It's time they started to use the spring in the north pasture. Then you won't have to worry about a water hole at the pond."

He gave no sign that he heard me but kept looking toward the pond.

"You know how much work it takes to keep a water hole open." He still was unconvinced. "Remember last winter how the cattle passed up the tub of water by the fence to go to the spring?" When he had the cistern dug, he had water piped to a no-freeze hydrant at the fence for emergency water in the north pasture for the cattle. Finally, he took the ax back to the tool chest in the barn, and we started to the house.

He had to stop four times to rest before we reached the back door. I had thought we could step into the tracks we had made coming to the barn but they were so hard to follow, we had to break a new trail.

As soon as we were inside, he changed to dry clothes and lay down on the sofa. From the expression on his face as he closed his eyes, I knew that he was surprised and disappointed that he was so exhausted. I shared his disappointment. He had seemed stronger for the last few days and I had thought he really was better.

That afternoon Dr. Trippe telephoned. "How's the snow out there?"

"Deep," I told him.

"I'm coming out," he said. "I want to see Ben."

"I would like for you to see him — ." Ben guessed who had called. He took the telephone from me and there was no mistaking his, "Oh-oh!" He could not have said, "No!" more emphatically.

When he gave the phone back to me he was still shaking his head. I had to explain to Dr. Trippe . . . "Ben is afraid for you to come. Your car could not get through the drifts in our drive. Let me call you after we get the drive cleared. I have had your prescriptions refilled. They came in yesterday's mail."

Ben went back to the sofa. He had won but he wasn't happy. I sat down beside him. "I know how you feel about Dr. Trippe," I said. "You don't want him to take any chances. Too many people need him."

He nodded and I could see that he was pleased that I understood. For a moment I was tempted to postpone telling him the orders Dr. Trippe had just given me. But he had to know. "Dr. Trippe says you are NOT to go to the barn until there is a big break in the snow."

He didn't answer and I said to myself, "He knew when he finally made it back to the house today that he would not be doing any more feeding for awhile."

Sorry as I was for him, I was relieved that I didn't have to worry any longer about his collapsing in the snow. As I started to the barn the next morning, I found myself zigzagging a new path. It was fun. I remembered the "fox tracks" we had made in the snow as children.

When I looked back and saw Ben at the window, he looked so forlorn, I stopped my foolishness. I knew that if I fell, he would forget doctor's orders and there might be two of us down in the snow.

The days that followed were much the same. Everybody in our area was snowbound for the first time in years.

One neighbor managed to clear his drive only to have more snow refill it that same night.

In ski pants and high boots, I made the trip to the mailbox every day. Christmas greetings from relatives and friends continued to come. The milkman and the bread man, who came once a week, chose the same side of the drive as I had. The snow was not as deep there as it was on the other side.

Groceries were no problem. We always kept a stock of staples. The freezer supplied meat, vegetables and fruit.

One day I looked out of the window to see our daughter Nancy's car parked just off the highway at our drive; and halfway down the drive came Nancy carrying two big sacks of groceries. Before I could pull on my boots to go to meet her, she was at the door.

My assurance over the telephone that we were all right had not convinced her. She had to see for herself.

By then it was doubtful that we would be able to go to their house for Christmas. It would be the first year we had missed since the grandchildren were old enough to enjoy Christmas.

When Nancy and Harvey insisted on coming for us, Ben was firm. Much as we wanted to be with them, he would not let them make two round trips, forty-eight miles, to come for us and to bring us back. Not only was our driveway impassable, but between our house and theirs were county roads with dangerous hills and curves, all snowpacked and slippery.

"All right," Nancy finally agreed. "If you can't come to us, let us bring our Christmas to you." Again Ben shook his head, and his "Oh!" meant "No!"

We celebrated Christmas alone, happy and thankful for our telephone calls and the Christmas programs over

2

radio and television. Never had we heard the story of the birth of the Christ Child more beautifully told. Christmas carols that we had loved since childhood brought back happy memories.

New Year's Eve was happy, too. From the year we were fifteen, we had not missed sharing New Year's Eve. First, at the watch parties at our church; later, we had always managed to be together, even that year when he was in service during World War I.

The day after New Year's was bright and warmer. Our driveway to the highway was still impassable but the path I had made to the barn was so beaten down, that when Ben pointed to it and then to himself, I said, "You want to try it?"

He did.

"All right. May I go along?"

He grinned and offered his arm. I saw the camera in his pocket and said, "I'll take pictures of you and BBM."

He was happy with the way BBM was developing. As he ran his hand over the calf's rumps, I could almost hear him say, "You're on your way, Champ."

Before we started back to the house, Ben wanted to go to the pond to see the water hole a friend had cut in the ice when he learned that Ben was worrying because he thought the cattle were not getting enough water at the spring. I had opened the gate to the back pasture, but Ben didn't want the cattle to go that far from the house.

I took two pictures of Ben with BBM and Rollette at the water hole.

On our way back, Ben stopped at the cabin. I had been watching for an opportunity to check the furnace oil in the tank. If the oil was as low as I knew it must be, I didn't want Ben to learn about it until I telephoned the agent of the oil company. The oil was even lower than I had feared.

As I took the oil measuring stick back to the basement, I saw Ben brushing off the fireplace grill at the cabin porch. I hurried into the basement. He must not see the tears running down my cheeks. What would we do if the furnace went out? The fireplace would be far from adequate. And how long would the logs last if we burned them day and night? The oven of the electric range wouldn't be much help. We couldn't go to Nancy's. Ben, even with help, would not be able to make it to the highway. We would be snowbound in a cold house.

"Dear God, what can I do?"

With the prayer, I grew calm. "Telephone for oil," I heard myself say, "before Ben comes in."

I ran up the stairs to the telephone. "The oil is so low the furnace may go out any time," I told the oil man.

"It will not go out," he assured me.

"But your truck can't get through the drifts in our drive. A man is coming today to clear it but he has only a small tractor. I don't know how long it will take him."

Never will I forget the oil man's answer . . . "I will get oil to Ben if I have to carry it down in five-gallon cans."

An hour later, Ben saw the man with the tractor stop at our drive, and motioned for me to come to the window. The tractor was even smaller than I thought it would be. How could it clear off all that snow? Why didn't the man get started? Was he afraid he couldn't do the job?

At last the tractor began to move. From the window, I couldn't see that it was making even a dent in the snow. It had gone perhaps twenty-five feet when it began to skid. I didn't know I had grabbed Ben until I felt his arm tighten around me. The man helplessly tried to stop the tractor as it skidded into the trench at the side of the drive.

We were still staring at the tractor when the oil truck stopped on the highway at our drive. We had not seen it come up over the hill. Five gallon cans, I thought; how many trips would it take? I hadn't told Ben I had called the oil company.

The oil truck pulled to the side of the highway. The driver was talking with the man with the tractor when we saw the highway snowplow stop at our drive. The man with the snowplow took one look at the oil truck and the tractor in the trench, then turned into our drive, hooked on to the tractor and lifted it, as if it were a toy, back to the drive. From there, the tractor moved to the side of the highway. Next, the snowplow came down our drive, sweeping it smooth as a ribbon.

Ben and I were still staring in wonderment when we realized the snowplow was moving back to the highway. Ben reached in the pocket where he usually carried his billfold, then apparently remembered he had left it in his chest of drawers in the bedroom.

When he went for it, I tried to stop the man on the snowplow. I called to him my "thank you" — and said that my husband was coming to thank him, too, but he waved and kept on going back to the highway. By the time Ben came, the snowplow was out of reach. We would watch for him and stop him the next time we saw him on the highway.

The man with the tractor came down the drive. He offered to clear a road to the barn. We were glad there was something he could do and we could pay him. It wasn't his fault he hadn't been able to clear the drive.

After he left, I said to Ben, "Now will you let me tell

Dr. Trippe he can come? Remember what he said about wanting to see you."

He shook his head and wrote, "I OK."

I knew from the way he was breathing he was not okay. Dr. Trippe must be called as soon as I could manage it without upsetting Ben.

He spent the remainder of the day on the sofa. That evening when I suggested, "Would you like to take your pillow and lie on the rug before the fire?" he shook his head. We spent many evenings on the rug before the fireplace, watching the play of the flames until they settled into a bed of glowing embers. That night he was too exhausted to enjoy the fire, yet he didn't want to go to bed.

It was after midnight when he went to our bedroom. Five minutes later when I followed him, I saw he was in trouble. He sat on the side of the bed, his face white and frightened.

"Won't you let me call Dr. Trippe?" I asked.

He nodded and I hurried to the telephone. In ten minutes we had a room at the hospital and an ambulance coming for us.

Still in pajamas, Ben walked to the sofa. I brought his clothes and offered to help him dress. He let me know he could manage, so I packed his bag, changed into a suit and slipped an extra blouse and sweater into the bag. When I didn't find my key to the house, I took Ben's key case from the top of his chest of drawers and dropped it into my handbag.

The ambulance arrived. Ben was ready in business suit, topcoat and hat. The driver took the bag and our little hand-operated emergency oxygen tank (Ben had let me know he wanted it), then asked Ben if he could help him.

Ben walked out of the house and down the steps unassisted.

The driver suggested that he lie down on the cot in the ambulance, but Ben took the seat that was next to the one that would be mine.

After I had closed the kitchen door, I saw I had not turned off the floodlights in the yard. The switch was inside the door. Not until I opened Ben's keycase did I remember . . . he had a new keycase. All his keys were in it and it was in the top drawer of his chest. Thank goodness! — There was an emergency house key in the cabin.

I hurried to the cabin, switched on the center light in the ceiling, went to the corner where the key was hidden back of a strip of building paper, reached for it — and dropped it. When I couldn't find it, I could only hope that Ben would not worry about the lights.

If he saw the lights as we drove away, he gave no sign. He handed me the oxygen tank and I kept it on all the way to the hospital.

It was wonderful to be greeted by a nurse who knew us. With her "Hi, Ben!" I relaxed.

A 24-hour oxygen tank was rolled to Ben's bedside. From the expression on his face, I knew how relieved he was. Had he been worrying all the time our driveway was drifted full of snow?

He was safe now. Back with the same around-the-clock nurses who had brought him through before. They would do it again.

14

Silent Victory

I sat in a chair at Ben's bedside for the remainder of the night. Yet without rest or sleep I was not tired the next morning. At last he was in the hospital receiving the care I had not been able to give him.

The sign on the door, "NO VISITORS," did not worry me. I couldn't believe his condition was critical. He had come through so many times before; soon he would be stronger and his friends could see him.

He slept most of the time . . . whether from sedatives or weakness, I didn't know. Sleep would help him to regain his strength.

It was late afternoon when he opened his eyes. As he looked out of the window I said, "I'll call a cab so I'll be home before dark."

He motioned for his tablet and pencil, and wrote, "KEY." When he gave the tablet to me, I caught a twinkle in his eyes. He had known all along that I had locked myself out of the house.

"I know where I dropped the key," I said, "I'll find it."

He pointed to the telephone. I was to call a cab and start for home at once.

"I'll find the key," I said again as I kissed him good-bye. "You'll know when I telephone you that I am safe inside the house."

He still looked worried. "It won't happen again, I promise. I'll put the emergency key back in the cabin and make sure I always have my key in my handbag."

He showed no improvement the next day. At five o'clock when Dr. Trippe made his second call for the day, I went with him to the hall and asked, "Do you think I had better stay here tonight?"

"It might be a good idea," he said. I thought he agreed because he knew I wanted to stay, not that Ben was in any real danger.

"I won't let Ben know I'm staying. He might think he is worse than he is."

I told him "good night" as if I were going home. From the lobby I telephoned Don, our neighbor, and asked him to do our feeding, then joined two other women who were spending the night there because they could not leave their loved ones.

The next night Nancy stayed with me in the lobby. Twice during the night we checked with Ben's nurse. No change.

The following night my brother and sister-in-law insisted that I stay with them because they thought I couldn't get the rest I needed in the lobby. When I wouldn't leave, my brother stayed with me.

Ben grew steadily weaker. Even the flowers and cards he always appreciated were unnoticed — all except the card from a friend who in the past year had suffered a stroke and aphasia. When his writing began to return, he wrote a card to Ben.

We spent one whole morning answering that card. Ben

let me know what he wanted to say. I wrote it down, Ben copied it and signed it.

Would he want this card answered? He did. I promised, "I will write today and tell him that you will write later."

He gave no sign he heard me. When he reached for his notebook and pencil I thought he was going to write something he wanted me to say. Instead, he wrote "CATTLE."

"Don (a neighbor) is feeding them," I said before I thought. Would he know that I was staying nights at the hospital because I couldn't leave him? I had been careful to keep the same hours I did when I went home. Apparently satisfied, he closed his eyes.

The days that followed showed no improvement. I tried to interest him in the newspaper and his favorite magazines. He would listen a few minutes, then drift off again. Nancy brought the book of poems they had read together. Before she finished the first five lines of "Abou Ben Adhem," Ben's eyes closed. We knew he was not listening.

Evening came that day before I realized it. When I saw Ben look out of the window at the fading sunset, I said, "Will you share your room with me tonight? It's later than I thought."

He nodded. I could see he wanted me to stay. Something in his smile, as he watched me arrange the pillows in my chair, made me wonder — had he suspected that I had been spending the nights at the hospital? Once, when I appeared earlier than usual, he had looked at his watch. Or was he just happy to have me with him? I wished I had managed it sooner.

I left the room only long enough for my meals (he insisted that I eat regularly) and to spend a few minutes in the lobby with friends who respected the "NO VISITORS" sign on his door.

When I returned from one of these visits, Ben gave me his tablet. He had written, "CATTLE."

"Don is still taking care of them."

He shook his head and wrote, "SELL."

"Shall I phone Art Adams?" He was the man who bought the other Polled Herefords and had told us to let him know if Ben decided to sell BBM and Rollette.

Ben nodded and wrote the price he wanted for the two.

Mr. Adams still wanted them and said he would come to the hospital.

Ben was pleased, but I guessed what he was thinking. "You want Mr. Adams to see the cattle again before he buys them?"

He did.

When I told Mr. Adams, he said he would come by for me that afternoon and we'd go to the farm.

BBM and Rollette came to the barnyard gate to meet us. "They look well cared for," Mr. Adams said. "How much does Ben want for them?"

I told him Ben's price. It was sometime before he answered, and I wasn't surprised when he said, "That is more than I can pay."

I named a lower figure. He agreed to it. I told him I would talk with Ben and call him.

Ben was watching for me. I think he knew what I was going to say . . . "Mr Adams still wants them but he can't pay more than — ." I quoted the price.

He looked out of the window and I knew how hard it was for him to cut his price. Finally he turned to me, held up two fingers, tried to snap the thumb and forefinger of the other hand and nodded.

"You mean if he buys the two right now, okay?"

He agreed.

As I reached for the telephone, I wondered if Mr. Adams had had time to return to his office. He answered so promptly, I thought he must have been waiting for my call.

"Your price is all right with Ben if you take them right away," I told him.

"Sold!" I reported to Ben.

There was relief and sadness in his eyes. I had the same mixed feeling. It was a moment before I could say, "You gave Champ (he smiled when I called BBM 'Champ') such a good start. Mr. Adams is pleased with the way he has developed."

He smiled again, then suddenly looked very tired.

The days that followed were quiet and peaceful. I sat beside his bed. There was no need for me to talk. He just wanted to know I was there and that I wanted to be there.

Once he pointed to Heaven. I knew what he was trying to say, but I couldn't speak. He pointed again and I said, "Some day, we both will be going." I still thought it would be "some day" for him, too. I know now he was trying to tell me — that for him it would be *soon*. If I had known, could I have said something to help? Was there something he wanted to tell me?

Two nights later, February 19, 1962, was like other nights. My pillowed chair was beside his bed. At nine o'clock, I said our prayer close to his ear, then touched my cheek to his. "I love you," I said. His cheek quivered in answer.

Shortly after midnight I heard the nurse speak my name. I will always be thankful she called me. I was beside Ben when he left us.

For Ben the stroke with its resultant aphasia was not the end, but a challenge. He lost his speech. He never gave up hope of regaining it. He lost writing. He practiced until he could print single words, often misspelled, but he kept trying until he made their meaning clear. His patience was amazing.

Life for him was a series of challenges. Goals won were lost when his heart ailment worsened. He settled for other goals that required less strength. Adjustment after adjustment — but always with hope and faith.

After his death, letters poured in from people telling what an inspiration Ben had been to them. The friend who after his stroke said, "Ben, you are a bigger man now than ever," was right. What more can any man do than inspire his fellowman to meet life's frustrations with hope and faith?

Appendix

LIST OF 1,000 WORDS
MISSPELLED BY BEN B. McBRIDE
AFTER HIS STROKE AND APHASIA

As the list indicates, there was no particular pattern in the misspelling. The most common mistakes involved omission, transposition, and the use of wrong alphabetical letters. Difficulty was experienced with short words as well as with long ones. Mr. McBride was unable to arrange words into sentences. Paradoxically, he could spell thousands of words correctly. He readily understood conversation and responded promptly with a nod, through a simplified "sign" language, or by printing a word or two.

Abou Ben Adhem......Ben Thou Abams
above.........................abouper
about.........................abuot
accident......................accidit
accuse........................assurd, accured
acid ....aidic
John Adams ....Adam
John Quincy Adams ..H. Q. Adam
advance ....avdance
ads ....adz
Aetna.........................Aenita
afraid........................afrade
Africa........................Arifca
after.........................afere, aftere, afore
against.......................asgant
agriculture..................arginista
Air Corps....................air crop

aircraft	araplianpe
alfalfa	alfalpa, alredra, atlafa, alfolda
algebra	abrerda
Alka-Seltzer	Alka
all right	arighter, aright
alone	alnoge
Alma	Arna
almanac	amlamker
ambitious	ambiouros, ambigion, amibuois
American Royal	Amerca Royar
Anderton	Anderer
Angus	Argus
another	anoughed
anthrax	anlixey
anticipate	anexpeneis
anxiety	anietxy
apology	apoyer
apple	apprilles
appliance	allgeneilce, allgentall
April	Apil
Arabian horse	Ribb Abia horse
architecture	archertica, arenertica
area	orea
Arizona	Azistano
Armour Packing Co	Aroumr Packer Co.
Arthur	Arurr
artificial	artcifi
artillery	arrellirey
artist	aritor
ashamed	ashamis
ashes	ashee, aeches

assessor ....accerice, accerrese,
                              asserise
Atchison ....Atsotha
athletic ....atlethic
Atlantic.....................Antinta, Anticta
atom...........................amot
atomic war.................atonic war
attitude......................allillide
auctioneer..................aicnetter, aicenttiener
                              (pantomined)
automobile ....auitombrole, auobomile
autopsy......................aurlosy, die
axle ....aexa
Ayres.........................Areys

bacon ....bocan
Ballard ....Ballrod
Baldwin.....................Balkink
banana.......................bannala, fruit
banter........................bantam
Baptist.......................Bishesh
barbed wire ....wire brareb
barrels ....brrl (drew picture)
Barry Church.............Church Berry
Bartholemus..............Banelanus
bathroom ....bafhroon
basement...................beatsantes, beastsan
Becky ....Bevky
Bearce ....Bearis
Behrens.....................Berin
Bells of St. Mary's......Mary, Holy Bell

Bertha ....Berha
believe......................beleive
believed.....................bevieled
Bernice......................Brenonsis
Beulah......................Belind, Bulah
B & G........................G & B
Bible..........................bilbe
bicycle ....bicykes
biscuits......................binknit
bitter ....bitting
black ....balck
blackberries...............blachbeerie
Blanche ....Blanhe
blanket ....bandit
blind..........................blinde
blizzard......................brizz
blue grass ....glue grass
blueprint ....bluid, plan print
Blue River ....River Blue
board..........................bourd, brored, boaret
Bob ....Bod
Bonnie Brae ....Bonnie Lee
bookcases..................bookceass
Bordeaux ....Beaxix, Beauxis
Boston ....Bolosh, Bostnos
Boyd ....Byod
brain..........................brian
Brazil..........................Brald
breath.........................bleache
Brenner ....Bermmer
Bricker ....Brinker
bridge.........................brirdge
bridle..........................brinll, bridt

brisket .... brister
broker .... boker, borker
brome .... groome
Brooklyn .... Broonlyn
brother .... brotred
brown .... bron
Buchanan .... Buchman
Buick .... Buirk
build .... bluil
building .... buiding
bulldozer .... drosser
bull service .... bull secine
bungalow .... bungala
Burpee .... Burhees
burlesque .... buqeske, buquake
Burlington .... Burangame
bus .... buss
bushel .... busher
business .... bussiness, businses
butter .... burturt
buttermilk .... burret milk

cabin .... bacin
cable .... calbe
calendar .... colamker
calves .... caver
camera .... carmere, camere
Campbell .... Cambell
captain .... captea
Carmen .... Cannen, Cermon
carpenter .... caperer

Caribbean	Carreban, Carebean
Caruso	Casurou, 13th Main (address)
cashier	casher
Cashier's check	Casher check
Caterpillar	Catepipner
cat fish	fish cat
Catholic	Cathelec
cauterize	acquoned, horse shoe, fire hoof
cement	cemtern, centret, cemoret, cemete block
cemetery	ceremenes
center	centren
central	certral
chain saw	wood chain
chains	chians, chains
chair	chiar
champion	chamtion
charcoal	colecate
chard	chacge
Charlotte	Charlrock
cheap	cheal
cheese	qurkard, clabber milk, creese
chemical	chemica, chemcal
Cherokee	Cherille
cherry plum	plum cherry
cherry wine	cheery wine
Chicago	Chigage
chicken	chichen, chick
children	chilern, child-ren
China	Chine

Chinese ....Chisene
choice.......................chioce
Christmas ....Christmes
church ....chruch
chute ....chuche
Cincinnati.................Cinnatti
Cindy ....Cinlly
cistern ....cramarsertern, cirtin
                                citsern, rainy water
                                (drew picture)
City Bond.................Bond City
city taxes 1962 ....tax city 62
civil ....civar
Clarence ....Clacene
Clay...........................Caly
Cleveland (city).........Clevevarr, Celeaced
Cleveland (Grover) ...Clevean
client ....clrient
Cline ....Cines
clock..........................clack
cloud ....cluod
cobmeal.....................meal rob
Coburn......................Curley
coffee.........................coffe
collection...................clloctinear
college.......................collerg
collie ....collier
Columbia College......Colurbia, Colinbia
                                College
commission 5% ....commist 5%
Communist ....Communrst
comprehensive...........compestrice, compasitel
concentrate................cerficar, certictration

concrete......................comtret
Confucian..................Cofuctric
Congress ....Cogress, Congres,
                             Comgress
Continental ....cintenal, contecal
consider.....................conrister
Consolivar.................Coversal
contract ....cancart, concert
contractor..................contacter
conventional..............contentional
Coolidge (Calvin)......Cooridge
corn crib.....................conr crid
Cottonwood River.....Cottowwood River
cough ....could
country.....................corty
Country Club ....Crotusoy
Country Gentleman...Gem Painlarr
county superintendent ..Superick Co.
courtesy....................cuestriry
crab apple..................applenck
cracked corn ....corn crack
crazy...........................crazing St. Joe
cream ....ceamer, cleam
credit..........................crebit
creek ....cheek
crib............................curb
croup..........................colees
cucumber...................cucummeker, cumbeuicin
Cudahy......................Cuhary
cultivator ....cuticator
curb...........................cibr, cirb, crub
curdle ....cucrebe
currant......................currat

curry comb ....horse brush
cyclone ....clymore, cyolone

daisy..........................diasy, daist
Dan Dinkle ....Dan Deintilce
damn fool.................Dafoll
daughter....................dauter, drater, Duather
Davis.........................Distern
dead man...................dieman (picture)
Dearborn...................Deerborn, Deardorn
deliver ....delevare, debvac
Democrat ....Domecrat, Demtracrot
Denver ....Dener
destroy ....dersoyer
determination............dermin—
die............................diad
Dierks ....Drerk
dillydally...................dittanery
disappointed..............misspoippitor
discount ....disount
distilled oil ....distern oil
distillery ....drillery
ditch..........................duth
dividend ....divided
divide ....divid
divorce ....divoeter
Dodge City................Doght (TV Wyatt Earp)
Domino Bull ....Dimmo Bull
Donna.......................Della
Dotson......................Diston
doughnuts ....doubuoy (picture)

Downing ....Doaning
Draftsman ....daltmerm
dream........................drean
Drennon...................Denne
drug ....durd, drud

Eckert........................Ekert, Ekrect
economics ....ecioncomics, ecomlict,
                          ecomticome
Edinburgh ....Enrgungruich
editor ....edonitir, editore
Edward.....................Ewdard, Ewdrard
Eisenhower...............Eisenhowes
Eldon ....Elbon
electricity..................electricy
elevator ....eelvater
Elliotts.......................Elliorts, 1513 Grand
                          (address)
Emporia ....Empass, Euplona,
                          Empaca
encyclopedia..............ecyredicia
engineering M U ....eignurgring M U,
                          errgrvagruic
England.....................Engand, Englan
English ....Ensli, Enlish
enigmatic..................eimitic
enough ....enuoch, enouht, enuold
entire.........................entile
equal ....uqualis, aequalis
equinox.....................eqinex
Erma ....Ernal

escrow ....Bond, extrao
Eureka........................Eurhekec, Eupeke,
　　　　　　　　　　　Erupeke, Eureka
exchange ....exhanlike, expnance
　　　　　　　　　　　(wrote 7 times, each
　　　　　　　　　　　different)
excited........................excita
exhausted ....exhaustired
expansion..................expnance
expense ....enpone
expire........................expnare
extra...........................extessas

Fairchild ....Fairturl
Fairmount ....Fahirmich, Faintom
family ....fimaly
fancy...........................framy, fracy
Farm Journal..............Joulam Farm
Faubion Co ....Fruetrung
Faust ....Fuarst, Devil
feather ....feater
February...................Februboy
Fence posts ....ferne (picture)
fertilizer....................ferisher, ferikr
fever ....fervere, ferfer, fever
FHA ....FAH
fiberglass ....glass Intera, figlass
fighter........................figter
Filger..........................Figler
finance.......................finace
financial....................finac

finish ....finfine
Firestone ....Fritsore, Firerose
Fisher ....Frrse
Florida ....Frotide, Frolida
flowers.......................frowers, forwer, frowler
flower seed ....fowler seed
flyer ....fryre
Ford ....Frod
Formosa ....Fosona
Fort Leavenworth ......Leaved
Fort Scott ....Frost Footh
Francis Bearce ....Franec Beares, Beasres
Frank Hart ....Hrant
Frank ....Frand, Yale
Frankie......................Frankey
freezer ....frezer, freezner
freshman ....frehsan, frshman
Friday........................Firday
friend.........................frieh
frost tonight ....frest—
fruit ....friut, fruft
fruit cake ....fruist cake
frustration ....histastisn, histation,
                                frst, fru....ion
fudge ....furgde, fungh
Fulkerson ....Furserke
furnace ....fura, furas

Gabelman...................Gatheman
Gadsden Purchase .....Gldlastome Purchurse
gap ....gop (out wire)

garage........................guage, garge, gargage
garden ....garten
garden snake ....gertan spake
Garfield.....................Gafren
Gashland...................Glasttone, Ganslang
gasoline....................gasonlene
Genesee ....Geness
Genesis ....Geniner
Genevieve.................Gevivet, Geneizeve
Gentry.......................Gnetry
George Tucker ....Geordge Turtres
George Washington ...Geoge Wash
Gladstone.................Gladlon, Glasltand
glove ....glore
Goldberg...................Golderg
Goodhue...................Guelhue
Goodyear ....Gooryear, Groohtry,
                          Groorhtyear
gooseberries ....greeseberries
governor...................gorgernt, govgermo
grader (road)............gravery, greader
graduate ....gruadiate
grandad ....dad gad
grandfather...............pa dad
grapefruit..................great pear
grapenuts ....gainde graindes
gravel ....garlvet, garlver
gravy ....gracey
grease.......................gecease
Grebe........................Gredies
Grecian ....Greese
Greek........................Greeck Greek
grocery ....gocelog, goclery, gregori

guinea ....gentian
gulf............................gupf, gufp
Guyman ....Guymor

Hagenah....................Hagneck
hail............................halt
halter.........................hatler, halter
hamburger.................hambricker, hamberger
Hamlet......................Hamel
Harding.....................Harting
Hardin Stockton........Stockern Harkok
hardware ....hardare
Harley ....Halrey
Harold.......................Halold, Halord
Hart ....Hrant
Harvey.......................Havrey, Havey
hasp ....hash (picture)
hayfork......................hayhaft (picture)
hazing.......................hazy
heart..........................hreat
heaven ....heaver
heavy.........................hever, hevel
hedge cheese ....hecedice
heifer.........................heiref, heifer
height........................heighet
Helen ....Hellen
Henry........................Henrhy
Herman Kuehlke.......Herman Kuekler
hereford.....................herefered
hickory ....hickey
high school................hiht school

highway	hiwardway
hinges	pirgee, hingle, himghing, hinghe
history	hickoyp
Hodson	Hosber
Holt	Holm
Home Builders	Buider Homes
hominy	honnica
Honolulu	Honuhuar
hope	pope
horse	hores
hospital	hospill, hositall, hostall
Hotel President	Hotel Presd
house	hourse
house plans	picta
Howard	Howad
Hoyt	Holy
humid	horrif
humidor	hominor
Humphrey	Humplery, Humphrey
hungry	hurgey, hurgary
hydrant	hyrant

idea	idion no (for no idea)
impossible	impossillip
income	imcome
independence	indencedence, indecdipence
Indian	Ididna
Indianapolis	Indionodalied
inflation	infalion

information ....informornorns
inspiration ....installion
insulation ....tresion, tecetsion,
                           inslation
insurance ....insuranise, insansican,
                           insuret
interest ....inrestest
Isham ....Isman
Israel ....Irseal
Ivanho ....Iovter, Ivanhoa

Jack Johnson ....Jach Jonhson
Jacques ....Kickness
Jefferson ....Jeffren
Jefferson City ....Jerfferen City
Johnson.....................Jonhson
Jonathan...................Johtson
Joplin ....Joplon
Joyce ....Jois
Judge.........................Jughe
Judge Southern ....Juthg Srothern

Kerosene...................Keserne, (distilled oil),
                           disternoil
khaki.........................kaika, khaki
kidney ....kindey
kindling.....................klinglish
knife...........................knefe, knife
kodak ....kokar, korak, koker, kokik

16' ladder ....16' lallerd, lethade
Lamplighter ....Lamptignor, Lamplichter
lariat..........................lartion
larkspur....................laspere, larpsure seed
lathes........................lathing
Lawn Acres ....Land Acre
lawyer.......................lawer
lazy...........................lazt, lase, lazey, tired
Leavenworth ....Leveater
lemon ....lomen
Lena ....Lene
lespedesia..................lezedia, lesredesa
lettuce ....lettice, lectuce
Lewis........................Lewen
Liberty......................Liberle, Librey, Librety
life insurance ....Lilf inviver
Lincoln ....Licnolle, Licion, Linlcon
Lindsay.....................Lighey, Lindasy
literature...................Lirtere
liver ....liven
locust ....Locuct
log chains ....chain log
Long Bell...................Londer Bell
Longfellow.................Long
lumber......................lumder
lunch ....luch
Lyon.........................Loyn

machete.....................messclicatte, Cuba,
                            messiltacetec, miceltate,
                            army navy store

machine	Machince
machinery	machinching
Maginot	Minagigetti
mallet	millen
manhole	(picture)
Manila	Minilla
manure	mamare, murale, manure
Man & Woman	man & wonen
Manhattan	Manttam
maple	magille
Margaret	Mareget
market	meraret
Martin City	Marin
Marvin	Maven
Massachusetts Inv. Growth	Massasuette Unvted
Mason	Marson
Maude	Maunde
Mayo	Maye, Mayo
mayor	moyar
McKinley	McKin
McPherson	McPerson
meadow	meahow
medicine	mecdid, medince, Ciba (name of pharmaceutical company with whom he placed salesmen through McBride Personnel)
Mediterranean Sea	Medianterninad (planning a trip for us)
Memphis	Mepriphes, Memken
Mendenhall	Merdalld
Mercy	Mecy, Mecry

Methodist ....Methist
metropolitan..............metrebran
Mexico ....Quexica, Newice
Milgram....................Milgrer
Miller........................Meller
minister ....misitere
Minneapolis...............Minnaepolles
Minnesota.................Mesrnecrate
minutes ....mutrintive
missionary................mieshioshiony, mission
                              miessevier, meissiarie,
                              China, 30 yr.
Missouri River ....Missoare River
mistake.....................miskate
mittens ....muntton
moccasin snake.........mocsinaces snake
modified ....molter
molasses...................molssas
money ....menoy, memoy
money talks..............$ talk o money
monkey stove ....mondey stove
Monroe.....................Mornon
monthly payments .....Mo. paymen
Morgan....................Morgar
mortgage ....morgage, morgation
motor ....moran
Muehlbach................Muellbach
music stand ....(picture)
mustard....................musarge

Nancy.......................Pancy

Nashua......................Nathvase, Nastus
neatsfoot oil ....greas liver
needle........................neetle, needle
negotiable..................negiated, negitio
negotiation ....negeviation,
                            noaeogesnagiat,
                            nogrogiaration,
                            nogrrargeatrion
Nelson ....Neslon
Nelle ....Nelley
Neosho River ....Neseop River
New Orleans ....Ne Orleen
Nichols......................Niclons
Nielsen......................Niesens
nitroglycerin ....glecreale
Nixon........................Noxin, Nixor, Noxen
Nolan ....Nalion
normal.......................nornan
novelties....................noxteles
nut ....nug
nurse........................nunres, nurne

ocean.........................sea, oceaf
October......................Octocle, Octonber
Oklahoma ....Oklameka, Oklmorlko
Olathe ....Olaelo, Otale, Othalhe
Old Rugged Cross.....Rigged Cross Old The
Oliver........................Ovilora
Omaha ....Omaho, Omalo
O'Neill......................O'Nien
onions ....oions

only............................onlk
opera..........................ofero
optimist......................opinist
options.......................opions
Orange........................oraneg
ordinary.....................ordinay
organ..........................ongral, ongerd (picture)
oriental rug................rug orientan, rug orental
original......................egruaver, egragrer
oriole..........................oricaile
Osage..........................Osago
Othello.......................Othero
(cold) outside.............(cold oustide)
oxygen.......................oxogon, oxyelye
Oyster........................oyeter, oyerhos

paddock.....................Barn portage
Paderewski................Parkinomis
paid............................piad
paint...........................piant
pallbearers.................mortayus, mogus
                             (picture)
Palomino...................Pamiedinia
paper..........................cepar
Paris...........................Piras
Parkview....................Parkvier
Parkview Hdw...........Parkview Hbw.
parsnips......................pasep
Paseo..........................Peareo, Paseo
pasture.......................partume, pasert
Patti...........................Perri

peaches.......................pecasses, pecaces
peculiar ....pecurian
pedigreed ....padad
peonies.......................peones
peony ....poeny
people ....peeper
pepper.......................panper
Percy ....Pecey
personality.................peslaaty, perpacter,
                           porpietpser (pointed to
                           Ike's picture and smile)
J. A. Peterson & Son ..L. B. Johsornson
petition.......................petiention, petetien
Phillips.......................Phipps
physics ....pyshic
physician ....pyhicans, Dr.
picking (corn) ....picknieg (corn)
pickle ....pickred, pictre
picture.......................pictcure
Pierce ....Piese
Pierson.......................Pieson
pigtail........................pigtighg
Pilcher.......................Picker
pineapple...................hipreappller
pioneer.......................pie
pitcher.......................pictice
pity.............................pila
plaid..........................prait
plan...........................paln, palm
planks ....planter
Platte.........................Patte, Platte
plow ....prow
plumber.....................plumbill

plumbing	ptumbing, plumping
plunger	plnebet
Plymouth	Pylometh
pneumonia	puelpuncque
poetry	poety
poison	piosne, piotson, kill
policeman	policyman
politics	polica, policatic
polio	plowre, plowle, ploler, Dr.
Polk	Plok
polled	polling
pond	poon
porch	porht
pork chop	polk
pork loin	pork lorn
Porter	Proter
possession	possesion
possible	possidible
post	posp
postcard	post crart, card post
posthumously	pressnlhush
potash	potasp
potato	totato
Powers	Powller
Prairie School	Prarie Schoorl 1905-1900 (he attended 1900-1905)
preacher	preahler
preserves	presesiue
president	predesident
pretty	pettrey
princess	pelles

print ....prine
printer ....prirther
procrastinate..............procinaticirn
proposition...............propievpion
prosecuting attorney..proctectre
Prudential.................Prudentian, Prudiature
pumpkin...................pkumkim
Puritan ....Peraitun
Purvis.......................Puris

quail ....quilt, qualt
quarter ....quater
quince ....quicne
quinine.....................quine, quiene

Rachmaninoff ....Richramros,
                        Reckinmitsic-piano
radiator ....reriantor
radio.........................rario
radish ....radice
rafter ....22 ft rooft
rake...........................rarke
raspberries.................racsberres
Ragland ....Roglan
receipt ....reciet
received ....recieved
refused ....refucded, refusded
register ....reginter, rersister,
                        rerrster

registered ....resisked deed
Rehard ....Reharb
remember................remineber
remembrance............remmustter
Republican ....Repuban
reservations ....rerevaseretion, ristation,
                          restivaction, restivetion
reservation...............restation, restivaction,
                          restiviction
residence ....residuce
restaurant ....rcaur
Rhinehart ....Rientaner
rice ....China
Richard....................Richard, OK
right ....righer
Riley........................Riney
rippling ....rittering, rippering
Riverside ....Rivedsere
roan..........................roen
Roanridge................Repore, church
Robert......................Robret
Rochester, Minn ....Rochecter, Min
rock..........................blade crush run, sbald,
                          slade, gnade
Roosevelt ....Roovllert, Rooveld,
                          Roovelt
rotary pump ....roratoy pump
round trip.................vp rount
Ruby ....Rudy
rugged......................rigged

saddle.......................Salldle

sadirons	saldi
St. Louis	St. Loost
salad	staded
salami	salaine, saugine
sales	slase
salesmen	slames, slasemen
salt pork	pork salt
Salvator	Salaherrutor
sanatorium	sarstory
sandwich	sambwich
Sarouk rug	Sessia rug
sarsaparilla	sasparilla
sassafras	sarsfras
Saturday	Satruday
sausage	saushice
sawdust	wood saws
scallops	scllopsep, scllandes
Schumacher	Schmanchnac
Schwarz	Swase
screwdriver	serws
secretary	sectreectray
security	sciocey, scivey, securt
senior	sermior, semior (senior)
sentences	sentnese
separate	seperate
service	sercive
Seven (7) up	up-7
sewer	sour
shady	showy
sharecrop	sharer, sharechopes
sharecropper	sharechopes
sharp	sprarpre
sharper	sreaper

sharpshooter ....plow-sweepleple
shed ....shep
sheep manure ....sheep mavin
Sheffield ....Sherffeed, Shefferd
shepherd ....sheperp
sheriff.........................sheffed, sherrife
Sherwin ....Sherinek
Shetland pony ....Sheffer
shiplap ....Lap barn, slap long
short...........................shorn
Shorthorn..................Shrothorn
shorts ....shords
shot............................shrock
shrimp.......................srinp
Shrine Hospital ....Shink Hotillatte
shrubbery ....shruegran
Siberian horse ....Seberians, Sibererian
Simpson ....Simpon
Sinclair ....Sinlair
skimmed milk ....skin milk
slippery ....sppisping
slipping ....spulping
smear ....screeher, calf
smell ....smeror, smeel good
smoke ham shoulder .smake ham shelder
smoky ....snomking
snow...........................sown
socket........................socking
soliloquy ....solollique, solilelique
sometimes ....somestand
sophomore ....soplormo, sorhorme
sorry...........................sorrel
sound ....sould

South America...........Americe South
South Dakota.............S. Dolakra
South Pole.................Scott Pole, scoocl,
                          Iceland Horse
Spanish ....Spansh
Spartan......................Strapt, Spirpa
specific ....specapetis
specification...............specapeticipie
spring.......................sping
Springfield.................Springfred
spring water...............sping water
square ....sprink
squash......................spuerke
squirrel.....................squrrel, spraigg, squilt,
                          srrinng
stakes ....(picture)
Standard Oil...............Stnodlnock, Stanlarn Oil
Staple ....slaster (picture)
state ....stane
statement...................stametsent
station ....saiton
steak.........................sreat
Stephens College.......Stephenes College
Stevens Ins................Sep
stirrup ....surep
Stockton....................Sothwell
Stockwell...................Sothwell
store..........................stask
Stowe Hdw................Hwd Stowe
strawberry ....starresberry
strawberries...............steebeebee
strawberry shortcake..stweebreey stord cake
stretcher ....strechrecher, strecharher

strike........................stirke, strite
Stout........................Stuot
sugar........................surag
suicide......................sucdice, sucicde, suidice
sultry.......................surely
summary....................snirray, sunnary
Sunny Slope..............Sun Surlpy, Sun Slopey
surgical.....................sugical
survey.......................serley
Sutton......................Sullan
sweet williams..........william sweet
swing........................sming
swimming pool..........sminles water
switch.......................snits
Swope Park...............Park Stwope
Syracuse, N.Y...........Sayrusky, N.Y.

Taft..........................Talp
Tannhauser...............Tannhaiser
Tastle.......................latter
taunt........................raunt
taxi..........................taxe
taxidermist...............Dr. taxistism
teacher.....................teaher, treacher
Teddy Roosevelt........Ted Rooveth
temperature..............temertorem, tem, terem
Texhoma...................Teramha, Texana,
                               Texahoma
Thanatopsis..............."Ho him whom—"
                               ("To him who in—")
thaw.........................tauf

theater .... thatcher, teater
thin .... tint
third .... thirld
thorobred .... treubrerd, proportion
Thorp .... Troup
thread .... thead
Thresher .... Theston
threshold .... thesdold
thrice .... trice
thumb .... tomls
Thursday .... Trusday
tickets .... tickick
tight .... tigt, tight
Timberlake .... Timrekerame
time study .... time sturdy
timothy .... timoy, timoh
tires .... trire
toggle switch .... snits
tomato soup .... tonatate soup
tomorrow .... tomorread, tomoriew
tonight .... tonigle, tonighy, nofinht
Topeka .... Tepeke
tractor .... trator
trading post .... trated
transmitter (radio) ..... trasinator
Transylvania .... Sylina
tree .... saw $hr?
Trimble Lake .... Trimmit
Trippe .... Trigg
Troost .... Troose
Truman .... Trman
Tuesday .... Tersday
Tulsa .... Tulse, Tusla

tumbleweed .... tumtolled
turkey .... turkes
turnips .... tirper, turtnip, turpin
turpentine .... tehtenrine, tirpather
Tuttle Ayres Woodward ...Tullwere
Tyler .... Tyril
typewriter .... twyhwrirlge
twisted .... twigehe

unadvertised specials .unavertised specils
uncertainty .... uncerteannty, unceited
uncle .... unatunca
understanding .... unstanthneh,
                           unstind sanbird
understand .... urderstand (circles his
                           ear)
unions .... uions, Hronffa (for
                           Hoffa)
United Fund .... Untied Fund
Unity .... Uinty
Universal Credit .... Uvinsel
usher .... uricht
Utica, N.Y .... Utai, N.Y.

vacation .... vaconentile
Van Buren .... Marvin Murren (for
                           Martin Van Buren)
vandalism .... vanlarg
vaseline .... valistren

veteran ....vetrean
vinegar ....veimegal
violin.........................vioiter, viotin, uiotin,
                            vioeler
vision ....unmms, unisuninvo

waffle.........................wallep
wagon.......................wagen
Wallington ....Wallimon
Walnut......................Waltid
Walt Whitman............Wellg
washer(bolt 1x5-16)..washser
Washington ....Washingon
watermelon...............melton water,
                            watenmelon
Waukomis ....Wormiksas, Wouthousic
weaned ....wellk, wealf, wealk
weather.....................watherr
wedge ....webb, web (picture)
West Point.................Pointer Wast
western......................wertern
Westinghouse ....Westingens
Westport Methodist ...Methost Wetsport,
                            Werprot
Weston ....Watson
What name? ....man nane?
whiskey ....whishey, whislery
whistle.......................whister
white ....wihite
white face ....wihle face
who else ....who etle

wholesale...................whowsale
Wichita ....Wichta, Wicita
Williams ....Willams
Wilson ....Wislon
will ....willis, willie, wills
wire stretcher.............sesterter, fenters,
                                  stripeer, streeseer
                                  (drew picture)
Wisconsin ....Wicskinsen
Witte..........................Willer
Wolferman ....Wolfaman
Woodland ....Wonlall
Writer's Digest ....Wretter Drest
14th & Wyandotte......14th Wytates
Wyoming...................Wymon, Wyominslge

yellow.......................yollew
yesterday ....yesday, yeserday

Ben B. McBride

... he won the silent victory

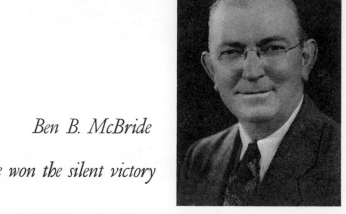

Ben B. McBride was born in Emporia, Kansas, the son of John W. and Mary L. McBride. The family moved to Kansas City, Missouri, when Ben McBride was in his early teens. He graduated from Westport High School in 1910, went to the University of Missouri at Columbia, and later attended the University of Kansas at Lawrence. He was a veteran of World War I.

Before his stroke in 1956, he was owner and manager of the McBride Personnel Service and president of Home Builders, Inc.

Mr. McBride was a member of Ivanhoe Lodge No. 446, A.F. & A.M., past High Priest, Kansas City Chapter No. 28, R.A.M. and the Kansas City Commandery No. 10, Knights Templar. Also, he was a member of Post No. 124 of the American Legion, and Forty & Eight, an honorary society of the Legion.

Before his retirement, he was a Shriner and a member of the Optimist Club, Kansas City. He was a charter member of the Kansas City Employment Board and a member of the National Employment Board.

He was chairman of the Platte County Republican Central Committee, and a member of Speakers 13, the alumni of Speaker's Training Courses of Advertising and Sales Executives Club, Kansas City, Missouri.

When aphasia stopped all these activities, Mr. McBride replaced them with others, most important of which was trying to help other aphasics.